COOKBOOK
TABLE OF CONTENTS

INTRODUCTION

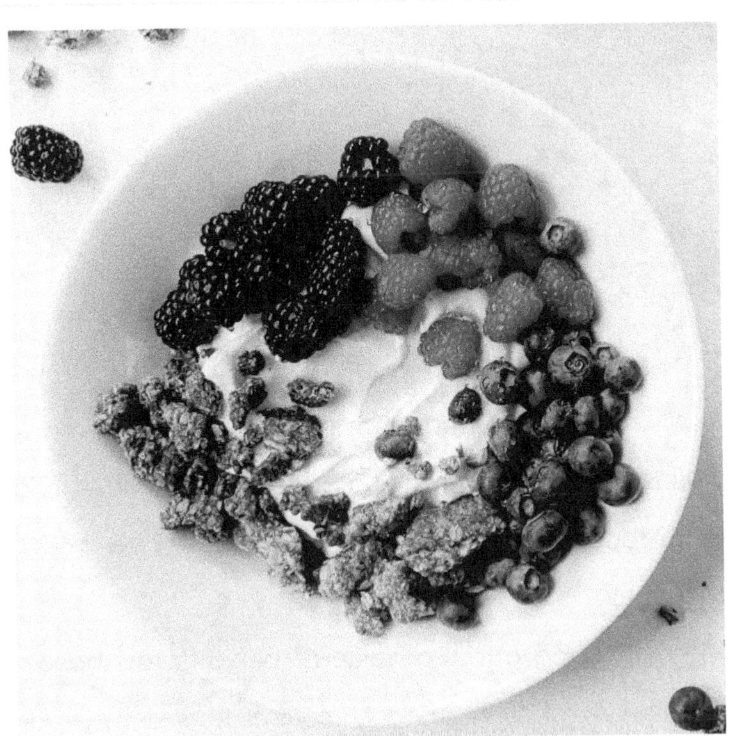

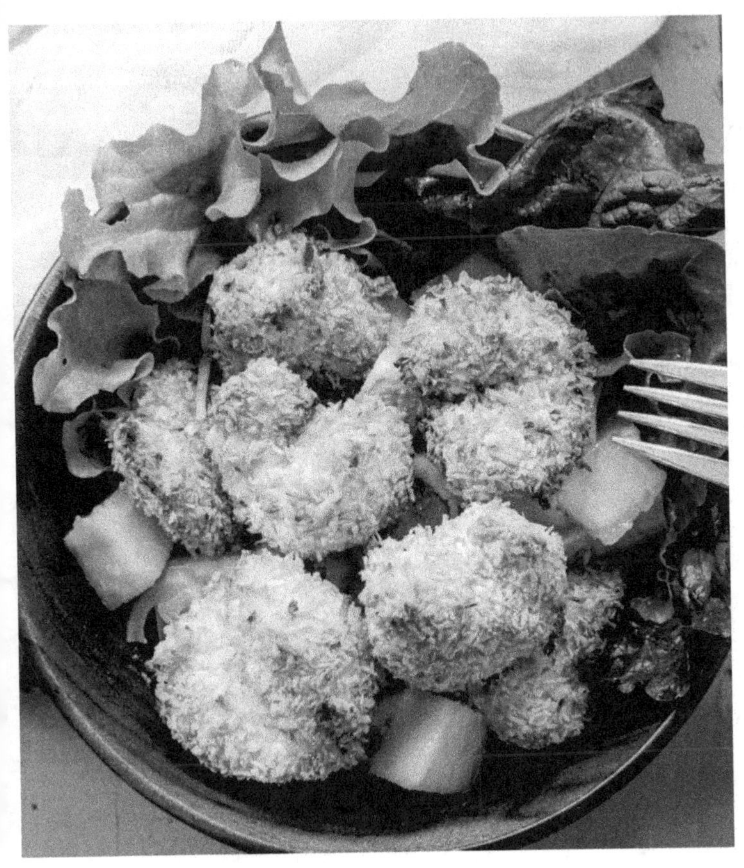

THE HEALTHY MEAL PREP COOKBOOK

In today's fast-paced world, maintaining a healthy diet can often feel like a challenge. Between work, family, and various commitments, finding the time to prepare nutritious meals may seem overwhelming. This is where meal prepping becomes a game-changer. By dedicating a few hours each week to planning and preparing meals in advance, you can save time, reduce stress, and make healthier choices throughout the week.

Meal prepping offers a range of benefits for those seeking a balanced lifestyle. It helps to eliminate the guesswork of what to eat, making it easier to stick to a well-balanced diet. Instead of reaching for processed, unhealthy options in moments of hunger or fatigue, you have ready-made meals that align with your nutritional goals.

Moreover, meal prepping allows for better portion control, helping you to manage your calorie intake and support weight management. By preparing meals ahead of time, you are less likely to overeat or snack on unhealthy foods. It also helps save money, as you're more likely to use ingredients efficiently and avoid the need for last-minute takeout.

Most importantly, meal prepping encourages mindful eating. It empowers you to make intentional decisions about the foods you consume and fosters a greater awareness of the importance of a balanced diet. With meal prep, you can ensure that your body receives the essential nutrients it needs to stay energized and healthy, even amidst a busy schedule.

In this book, we aim to simplify the meal prep process, providing you with easy-to-follow recipes, tips, and meal planning strategies that make preparing healthy meals effortless and enjoyable. By adopting meal prep into your routine, you'll find it easier to maintain a healthy lifestyle, stay organized, and nourish your body with wholesome, delicious food every day.

Common Challenges of Not Having a Meal Plan and How Meal Prep Solves Them

Without a proper meal plan, it's easy to fall into the trap of unhealthy eating habits. Many people struggle with making nutritious choices when they're pressed for time or unsure of what to prepare. This often leads to impulsive decisions like grabbing fast food, skipping meals, or relying on processed snacks—none of which support long-term health. Additionally, the lack of planning can create stress and frustration, as you may find yourself scrambling to put together a meal at the last minute.

Meal prep is a powerful solution to these challenges. By planning and preparing meals in advance, you eliminate the stress of daily meal decisions. Having ready-made meals on hand ensures that you're fueling your body with the right nutrients, even when you're short on time. Meal prep also reduces the temptation to rely on unhealthy options, as you'll have healthier meals conveniently prepared and waiting for you.

The Importance of a Balanced and Consistent Diet

Eating a balanced and consistent diet is essential for maintaining optimal health. A well-rounded diet provides your body with the necessary vitamins, minerals, and nutrients to function properly, boost energy, and prevent chronic diseases. When meals are haphazard and inconsistent, it's harder to meet your nutritional needs, which can lead to fatigue, poor concentration, and long-term health issues.

Meal prepping makes it easier to maintain balance in your diet. By taking time to plan meals ahead, you can ensure each meal includes a variety of food groups, delivering essential nutrients for a healthy lifestyle. Consistent, nutritious eating also stabilizes blood sugar levels, improves digestion, and promotes overall well-being.

The Goal of This Book

The goal of this book is to help you simplify the process of organizing and preparing healthy meals for your daily routine. We aim to take the guesswork out of meal planning by offering practical, easy-to-follow recipes and meal prep strategies. With the guidance provided here, you'll be able to create balanced, wholesome meals that support your health goals and fit seamlessly into your lifestyle. Whether you're a beginner or an experienced cook, this book will make it easier for you to establish a sustainable meal prep routine that leads to better eating habits and a healthier life.

What is Meal Prep? Definition and Reasons to Apply It

Meal prep, short for meal preparation, is the process of planning, preparing, and often cooking your meals in advance. This could involve making entire meals ahead of time or simply preparing ingredients in bulk to make cooking easier during the week. The primary goal of meal prep is to save time, reduce stress, and ensure you always have healthy, balanced meals on hand, even when life gets busy. By setting aside a specific time to plan and cook, you eliminate the need for last-minute decisions about what to eat, which often leads to unhealthy choices.

There are several reasons why meal prep is beneficial:

- **Time-saving:** Preparing meals in advance allows you to avoid the daily task of cooking, giving you more free time during the week.
- **Healthier eating:** With meal prep, you can control the ingredients and portions, ensuring that your meals are nutritious and balanced.
- **Money-saving:** Planning meals helps you avoid unnecessary food purchases and reduces food waste by only buying what you need.
- **Less stress:** With meals prepared ahead, there's no more worrying about what to cook when you're busy or tired.

Basic Steps to Prepare Meals in Advance: From Planning to Cooking

1. **Planning:** The first step in meal prepping is to plan your meals for the week. Consider your schedule, dietary goals, and food preferences. Create a menu that includes a balance of protein, vegetables, healthy fats, and whole grains.
2. **Shopping:** Once you have a plan, make a grocery list of all the ingredients you'll need. Sticking to the list helps prevent impulse buys and ensures you have everything ready for the week.
3. **Prepping:** After grocery shopping, start the meal prep process by washing, chopping, and portioning ingredients. You can also cook certain items in bulk, like grains or proteins, to make meal assembly quicker during the week.
4. **Cooking:** Depending on your preference, you can cook entire meals and store them for the week, or simply prepare ingredients to be quickly assembled into dishes. Make sure to portion meals appropriately and store them in the refrigerator or freezer.

Essential Tools for Meal Prep

Having the right tools can make meal prep much easier and more efficient. Here are some key items you might need:

- **Storage Containers:** Airtight containers are essential for storing prepped meals and ingredients. Choose ones that are microwave-safe and come in a variety of sizes for different portions.
- **Food Scale:** A food scale helps you measure portions accurately, ensuring your meals are balanced and meet your dietary needs.
- **Pressure Cooker or Slow Cooker:** These appliances are great for cooking in bulk, allowing you to prepare large quantities of food without much effort.
- **Knife Set and Cutting Board:** Good-quality knives and a sturdy cutting board make chopping and slicing ingredients faster and safer.
- **Meal Prep Bags:** Insulated meal prep bags or lunch boxes are perfect for taking your prepped meals on the go.

Smart Meal Planning: How to Create a Weekly Menu

Effective meal prep starts with smart meal planning. Here's how you can create a weekly menu:

1. **Assess Your Needs:** Consider how many meals you'll need each day and for how many people. Take into account any upcoming events or busy days where quick meals will be necessary.
2. **Balance Your Meals:** Make sure each meal includes a balance of protein, carbs, fats, and fiber. Variety is key to keeping your diet interesting and nutritious.
3. **Batch Cooking:** Plan meals that allow for batch cooking. This way, you can make larger portions of certain dishes and eat them throughout the week, reducing overall cooking time.
4. **Incorporate Versatile Ingredients:** Choose ingredients that can be used in multiple meals. For example, a large batch of roasted vegetables can be used in salads, wraps, or as side dishes.
5. **Create a Schedule:** Decide which day of the week will be your meal prep day. Organize your cooking tasks to maximize efficiency, such as roasting vegetables while boiling grains or cooking proteins simultaneously.

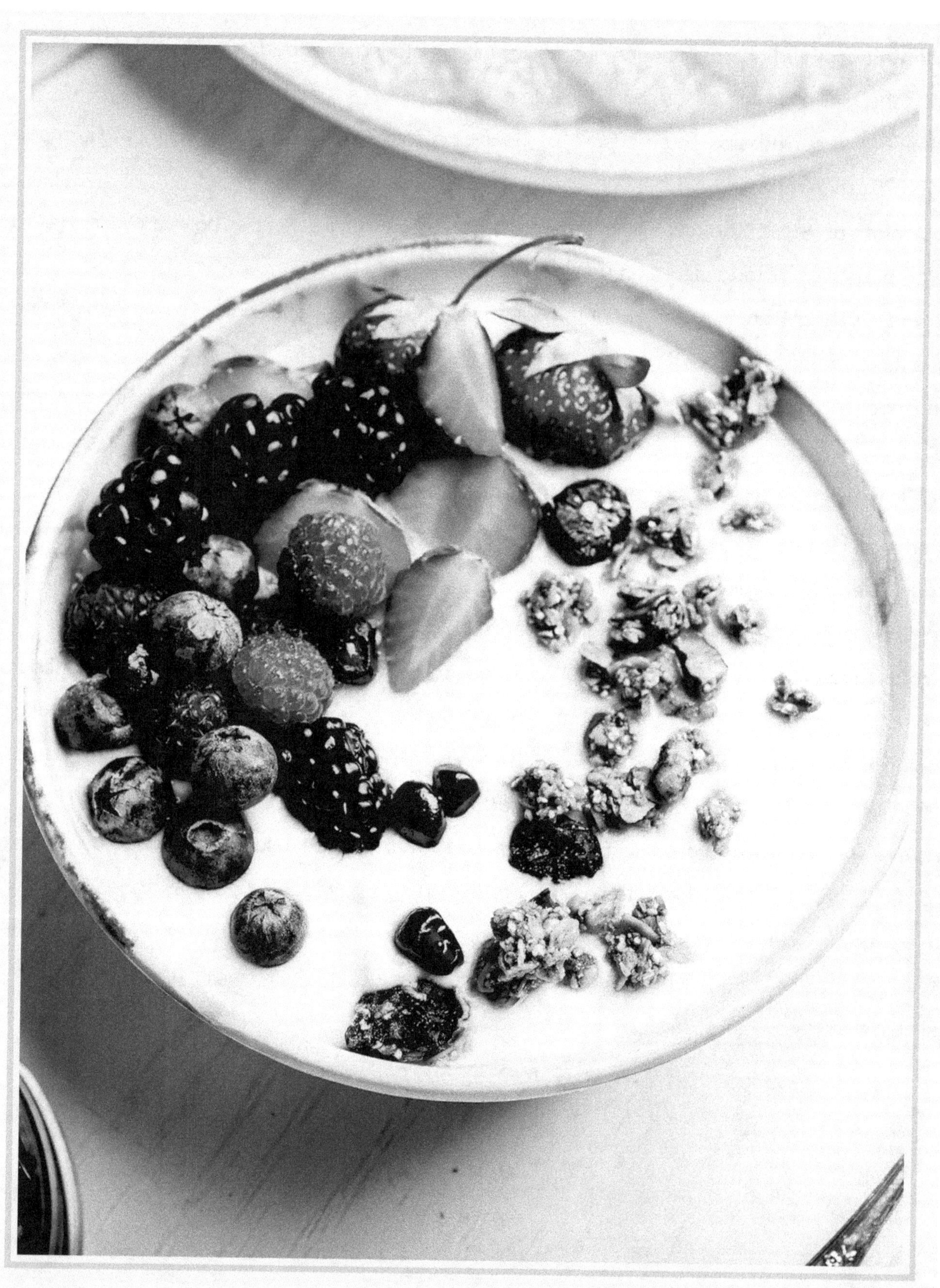

TABLE OF CONTENTS

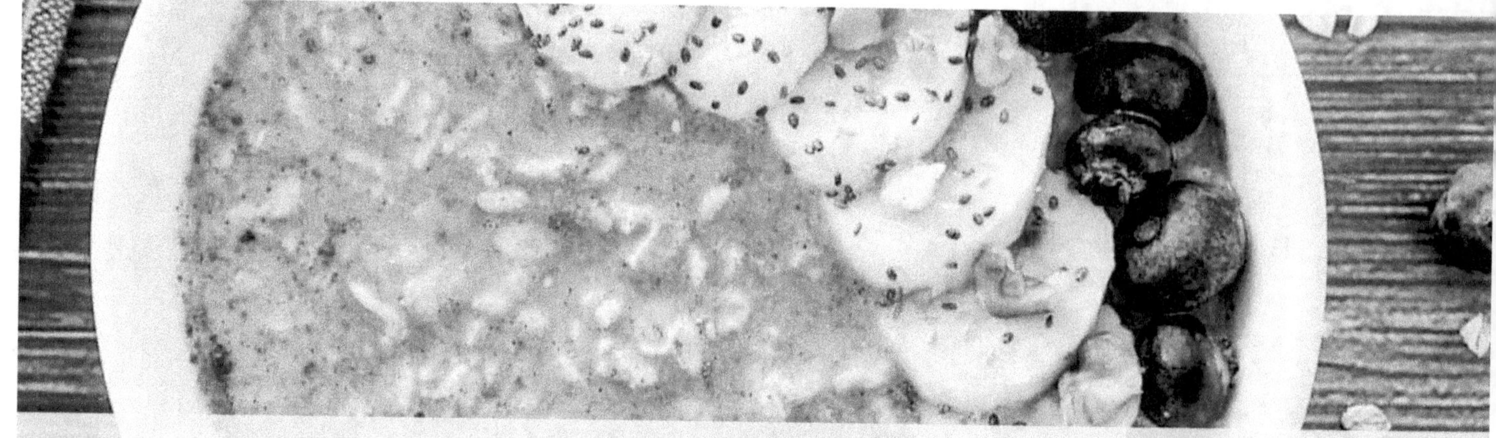

OVERNIGHT OATS WITH BANANA AND CHIA SEEDS

This delicious and nutritious Overnight Oats recipe is a perfect way to kickstart your day with a healthy meal prep option. Packed with fiber-rich oats, chia seeds, and the natural sweetness of banana, this make-ahead breakfast will keep you full and energized throughout the morning. It's ideal for a quick grab-and-go meal.

Serves	 **Preparation Time**		**Cooking Time**	
4	10 minutes		0 minute	

Ingredients:

2 cups rolled oats

2 tbsp chia seeds

2 cups almond milk (or any milk of choice)

2 ripe bananas, sliced

1 tbsp sucralose (optional, for sweetness)

1 tsp vanilla extract

Fresh berries or nuts for topping (optional)

Instructions:

1. **Combine Ingredients:** In a large bowl or jar, mix the rolled oats, chia seeds, and almond milk. Stir well to combine.
2. **Add Flavorings:** Stir in the vanilla extract and honey or maple syrup if using. Add a pinch of cinnamon if desired.
3. **Add Bananas:** Gently fold in the sliced bananas, distributing them evenly throughout the mixture.
4. **Refrigerate:** Cover the bowl or jar with a lid or plastic wrap. Refrigerate overnight, or for at least 6 hours, to allow the oats and chia seeds to absorb the liquid and soften.
5. **Serve:** In the morning, give the oats a good stir. If the mixture is too thick, add a little more milk to reach your desired consistency. Serve cold and enjoy!

Nutrients (per serving)

Calories: 210 kcal Carbohydrates: 40g Fiber: 6g

Protein: 5g Fat: 4g Sugar: 7g Sodium: 60mg

Calcium: 120mg

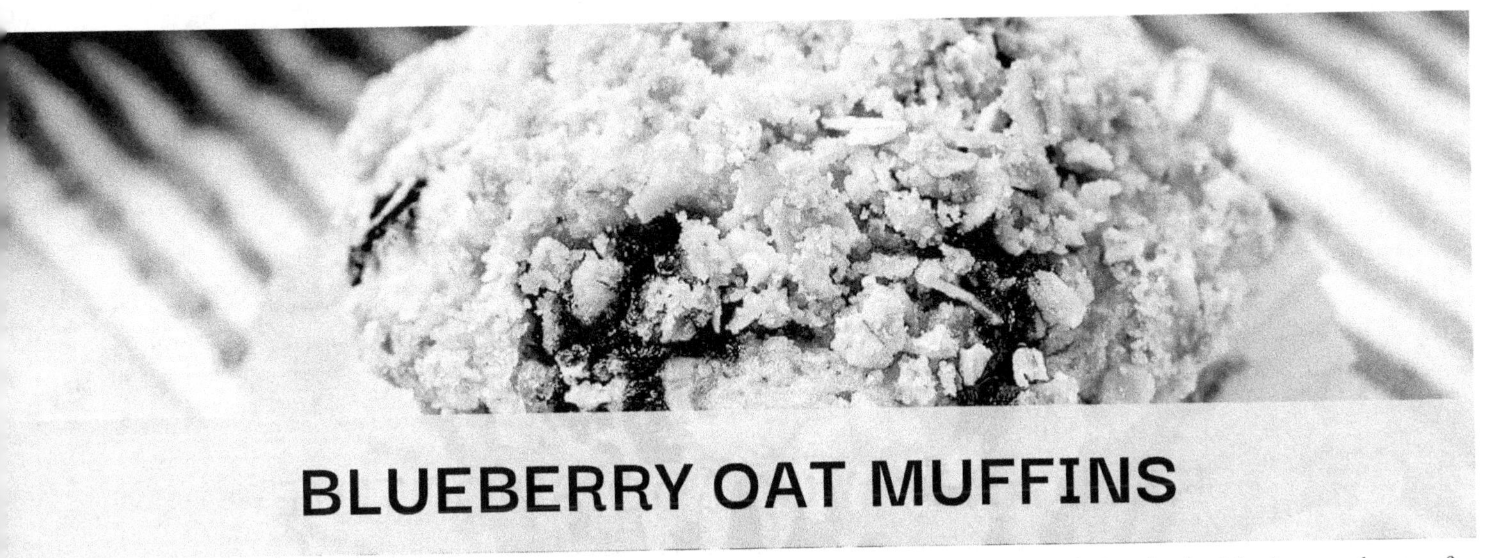

BLUEBERRY OAT MUFFINS

Blueberry Oat Muffins are a perfect healthy meal prep option for breakfast or a snack. Packed with the goodness of whole oats and fresh blueberries, these muffins are naturally sweetened with sucralose, making them a delicious and nutritious treat that's easy to prepare ahead of time.

Serves		Preparation Time		Cooking Time	
4		15 minutes		20 minute	

Ingredients:

2 cups fresh kale leaves (stems removed)

1 ripe avocado

1 ½ cups unsweetened almond milk (or milk of choice)

1 tbsp sucralose

1 small banana

1 tbsp chia seeds

1 tsp vanilla extract

1 cup ice cubes

Instructions:

1. **Add Ingredients:** Add the fresh kale leaves, avocado, almond milk, banana, and sucralose to a blender.
2. **Blend Smoothly:** Blend on high speed until smooth and creamy.
3. **Combine Extras:** Add the chia seeds, vanilla extract, and ice cubes, and blend again until well combined and chilled.
4. **Taste and Adjust:** Taste and adjust sweetness or thickness by adding more sucralose or almond milk if needed.
5. **Serve:** Pour into glasses and enjoy immediately, or refrigerate for up to 24 hours.

Nutrients (per serving)

Calories: 170 kcal Carbohydrates: 16g Fiber: 6g

Protein: 4g Fat: 10g Sugar: 5g Sodium: 120mg

Calcium: 180mg

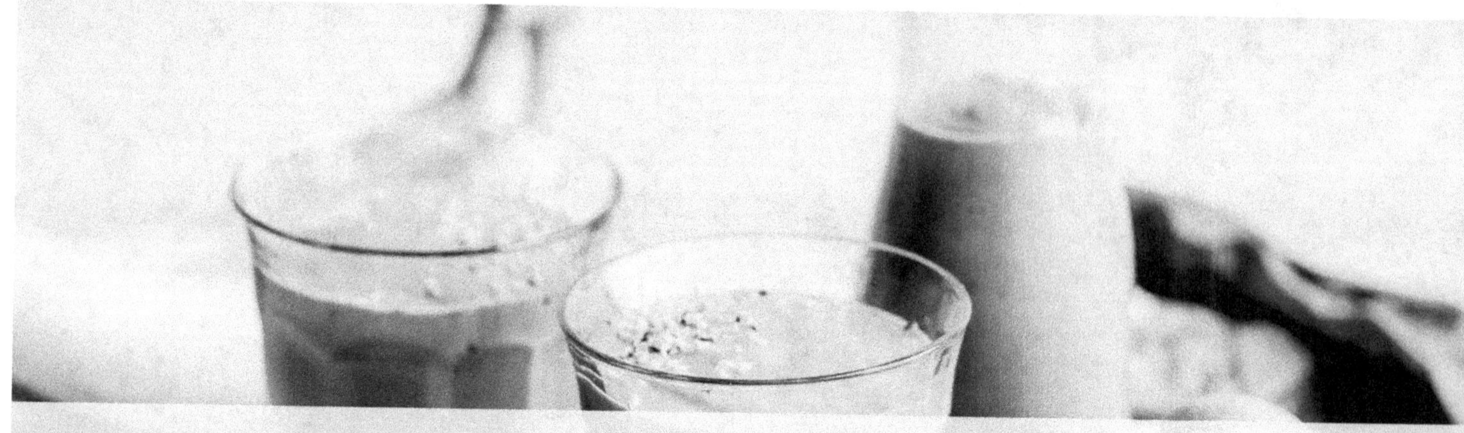

KALE AND AVOCADO SMOOTHIE

This Kale and Avocado Smoothie is a creamy, nutrient-packed drink perfect for a healthy meal prep. Loaded with vitamins, healthy fats, and fiber, this smoothie is a great way to fuel your body while keeping you full and energized throughout the day. Naturally sweetened with sucralose, it's both refreshing and satisfying.

Serves 	**Preparation Time** 	**Cooking Time** 
4	10 minutes	0 minute

Ingredients:

1 cup plain Greek yogurt (low-fat or fat-free)
1/2 cup mixed berries (strawberries, blueberries, raspberries)
1 tablespoon chia seeds
1 tablespoon honey or maple syrup (optional, to taste)
1/2 teaspoon vanilla extract (optional)

Instructions:

1. **Prepare the Yogurt:** In a bowl, mix the Greek yogurt with honey or maple syrup and vanilla extract if using. Stir until well combined.
2. **Assemble the Dish:** Spoon the yogurt into a serving bowl. Top with mixed berries and sprinkle with chia seeds.
3. **Serve:** Enjoy immediately as a refreshing and healthy breakfast or snack.

Nutrients (per serving)

Calories: 180 Sodium: 60 mg Carbohydrates: 24 g
Fiber: 5 g Protein: 13 g Calcium: 150 mg Fat: 5 g
Sugar: 15 g

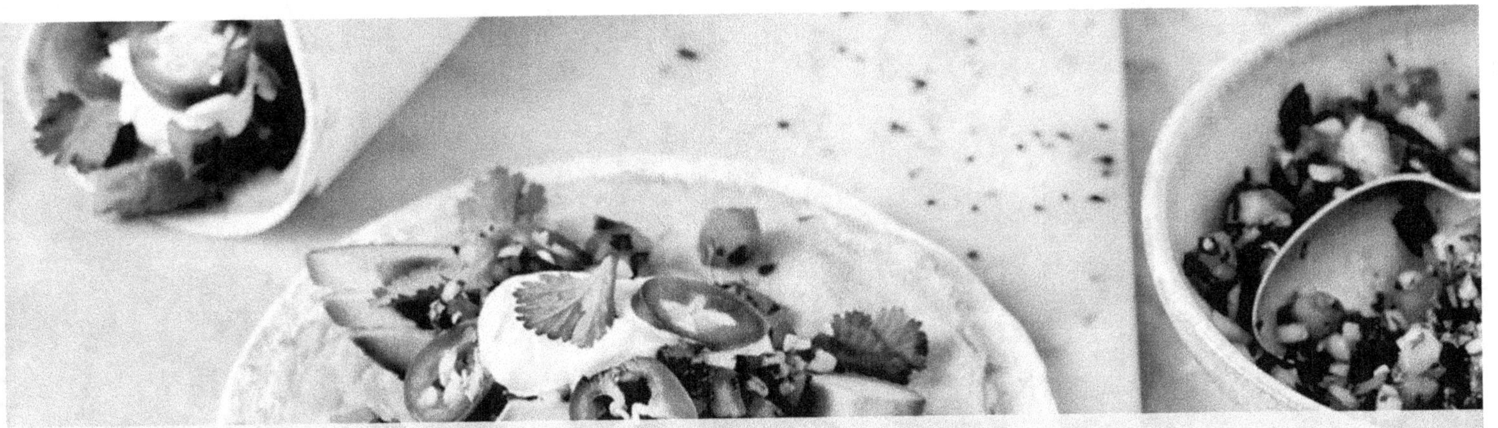

VEGGIE OMELETTE WRAPS

These Veggie Omelette Wraps are a healthy and convenient meal prep option, perfect for breakfast or lunch. Packed with fresh vegetables, eggs, and wrapped in a whole-grain tortilla, this dish provides a balanced mix of protein, fiber, and essential vitamins to keep you energized throughout the day. Lightly sweetened with sucralose, they offer a flavorful and guilt-free meal.

Serves	Preparation Time	Cooking Time
4	5 minutes	2 minute

Ingredients:

- 8 large eggs
- 1 cup diced bell peppers (any color)
- 1 cup spinach leaves
- 1 small onion, finely chopped
- 1/2 cup shredded low-fat cheese
- 1 tsp sucralose
- 1 tbsp olive oil
- Salt and pepper to taste
- 4 whole-grain tortillas

Instructions:

1. **Whisk Eggs:** In a bowl, whisk the eggs, sucralose, salt, and pepper together.
2. **Sauté Vegetables:** Heat olivo oil in a large non-stick pan over medium heat. Add chopped onions and bell peppers, and sauté for 3-4 minutes until softened.
3. **Add Spinach:** Add the spinach and cook for an additional 2 minutes until wilted.
4. **Scramble Eggs:** Pour the egg mixture into the pan and scramble the eggs with the vegetables. Stir occasionally until fully cooked, about 5-7 minutes.
5. **Add Cheese:** Remove from heat and stir in the shredded cheese until melted and well combined.
6. **Prepare Wraps:** Warm the whole-grain tortillas and divide the omelette mixture evenly among them. Roll each tortilla tightly, folding in the sides to create wraps.
7. **Serve or Store:** Serve immediately, or wrap in foil and refrigerate for meal prep.

Nutrients (per serving)

Calories: 250 kcal Carbohydrates: 18g Fiber: 5g

Protein: 16g Fat: 12g Sugar: 3g Sodium: 390mg

Calcium: 150mg

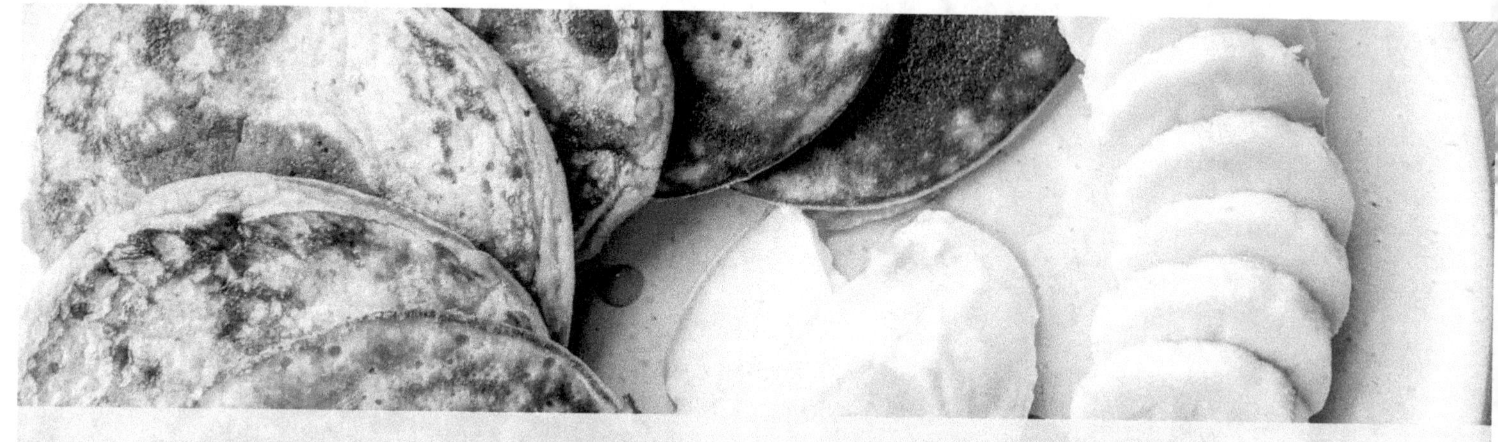

PROTEIN PANCAKES

Protein Pancakes are the perfect way to kickstart your day with a healthy, filling breakfast. Packed with high-protein ingredients and lightly sweetened with sucralose, these pancakes will satisfy your cravings without the extra sugar. They are ideal for meal prep and can be enjoyed throughout the week for a nutritious breakfast or snack.

Serves		**Preparation Time**		**Cooking Time**	
4		5 minutes		10 minute	

Ingredients:

1 cup rolled oats
1 scoop vanilla protein powder
2 large eggs
1/2 cup Greek yogurt
1/2 cup almond milk
1 tsp sucralose
1 tsp vanilla extract
1/2 tsp baking powder
1/4 tsp cinnamon
Olive oil spray for cooking

Instructions:

1. **Blend Ingredients:** In a blender, combine rolled oats, protein powder, eggs, Greek yogurt, almond milk, sucralose, vanilla extract, baking powder, and cinnamon. Blend until smooth and well combined.
2. **Heat Skillet:** Heat a non-stick skillet over medium heat and lightly coat with olive oil spray.
3. **Cook Pancakes:** Pour 1/4 cup of the batter onto the skillet for each pancake. Cook for 2-3 minutes, or until bubbles form on the surface, then flip and cook for another 1-2 minutes until golden brown.
4. **Repeat Cooking:** Repeat with the remaining batter, adding more oil spray as needed.
5. **Serve:** Serve warm with your favorite toppings such as fresh berries, Greek yogurt, or a drizzle of sugar-free syrup.

Nutrients (per serving)

Calories: 210 kcal Carbohydrates: 22g Fiber: 4g

Protein: 15g Fat: 5g Sugar: 2g Sodium: 180mg

Calcium: 120mg

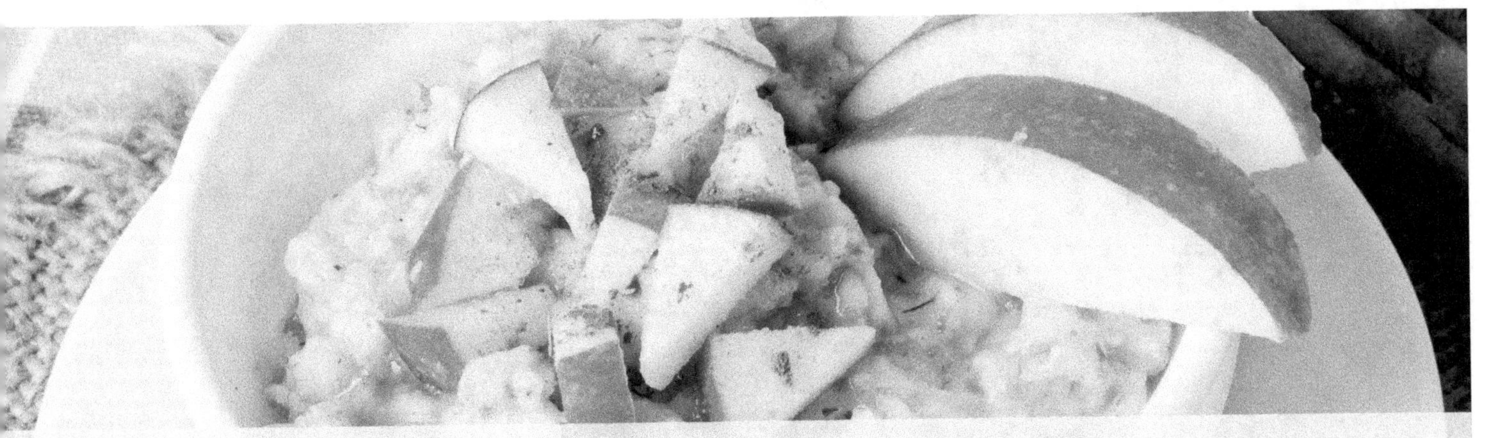

APPLE CINNAMON OATMEAL

Apple Cinnamon Oatmeal is a comforting and nutritious breakfast that's perfect for meal prep. This recipe combines the natural sweetness of apples with the warm spice of cinnamon and is lightly sweetened with sucralose. It's an ideal way to start your day with a wholesome, fiber-rich meal that will keep you satisfied and energized.

Serves 	**Preparation Time**	**Cooking Time** 
4	10 minutes	20 minute

Ingredients:

- 1 cup rolled oats
- 2 cups water or almond milk
- 1 medium apple, peeled, cored, and diced
- 1/4 cup sucralose
- 1 tsp ground cinnamon
- 1/4 tsp ground nutmeg
- 1/4 tsp salt
- 1 tbsp chopped walnuts (optional)
- 1 tbsp raisins or dried cranberries (optional)

Instructions:

1. **Boil Liquid:** In a medium saucepan, bring water or almond milk to a boil.
2. **Add Oats:** Add the rolled oats and reduce heat to a simmer. Cook for 5 minutes, stirring occasionally.
3. **Incorporate Flavors:** Add the diced apple, sucralose, cinnamon, nutmeg, and salt. Stir well to combine.
4. **Simmer:** Continue to simmer for an additional 10-15 minutes, or until the oats are tender and the mixture has thickened to your desired consistency.
5. **Add Toppings:** Stir in walnuts and raisins or dried cranberries, if using.
6. **Serve:** Serve warm, and top with additional apple slices or a drizzle of almond milk if desired.

Nutrients (per serving)

Calories: 180 kcal Carbohydrates: 30g Fiber: 4g

Protein: 4g Fat: 3g Sugar: 8g Sodium: 150mg

Calcium: 90mg

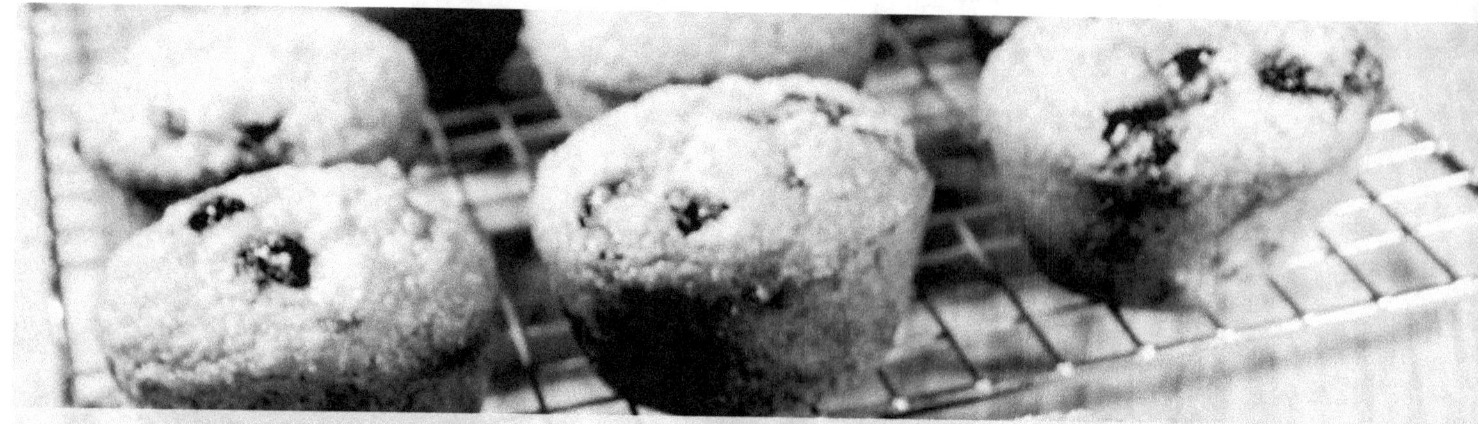

ALMOND FLOUR BREAKFAST MUFFINS

Almond Flour Breakfast Muffins are a fantastic option for a quick, healthy breakfast that's both low in carbs and rich in protein. These muffins are naturally sweetened with sucralose and packed with the goodness of almond flour, making them a perfect choice for a nutritious, energy-boosting start to your day. They're ideal for meal prep and can be enjoyed on the go!

Serves	Preparation Time	Cooking Time
12	10 minutes	25 minute

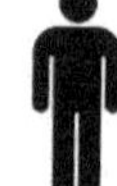

Ingredients:

2 cups almond flour
1/4 cup sucralose
1/2 tsp baking powder
1/4 tsp salt
3 large eggs
1/4 cup melted coconut oil
1/2 cup unsweetened applesauce
1 tsp vanilla extract
1/2 cup blueberries or chopped nuts (optional)

Instructions:

1. **Preheat Oven:** Preheat the oven to 350°F (175°C). Line a muffin tin with paper liners or lightly grease it.
2. **Mix Dry Ingredients:** In a large bowl, combine almond flour, sucralose, baking powder, and salt.
3. **Combine Wet Ingredients:** In another bowl, whisk together eggs, melted coconut oil, applesauce, and vanilla extract.
4. **Combine Mixtures:** Pour the wet ingredients into the dry ingredients and mix until well combined.
5. **Fold in Add-ins:** Gently fold in blueberries or nuts, if using.
6. **Fill Muffin Cups:** Divide the batter evenly among the 12 muffin cups.
7. **Bake:** Bake for 20-25 minutes, or until a toothpick inserted into the center of a muffin comes out clean.
8. **Cool:** Allow muffins to cool in the tin for 5 minutes, then transfer to a wire rack to cool completely.

Nutrients (per serving)

Calories: 150 kcal Carbohydrates: 8g Fiber: 3g
Protein: 6g Fat: 12g Sugar: 1g Sodium: 150mg
Calcium: 100mg

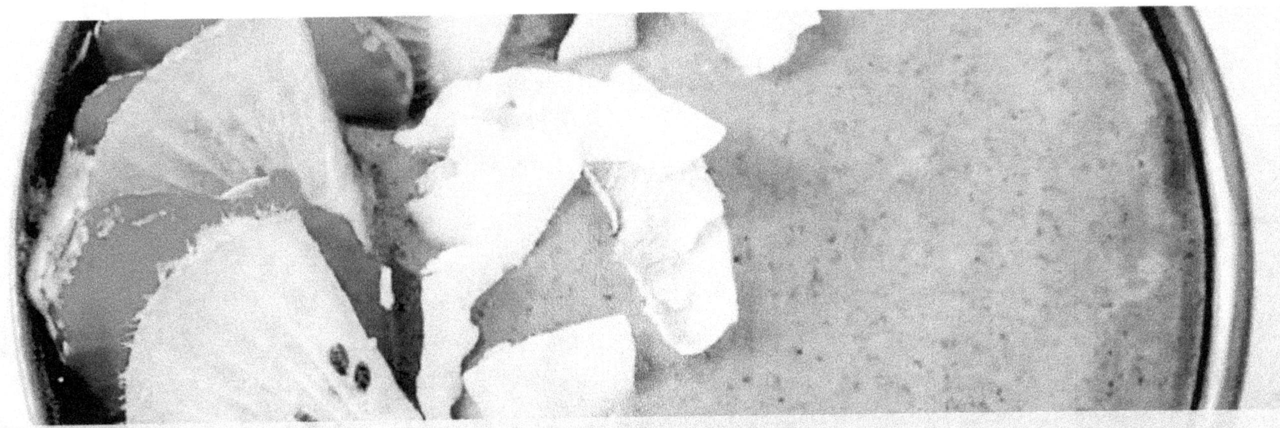

STRAWBERRY FLAXSEED SMOOTHIE

The Strawberry Flaxseed Smoothie is a refreshing and nutritious drink that's perfect for a quick breakfast or a healthy snack. Packed with the antioxidants of strawberries and the omega-3 fatty acids from flaxseeds, this smoothie is naturally sweetened with sucralose, making it both delicious and diet-friendly. It's an excellent way to start your day or re-energize in the afternoon.

Serves		Preparation Time		Cooking Time	
2		5 minutes		0 minute	

Ingredients:

1 cup fresh or frozen strawberries

1 tablespoon flaxseeds

1/2 cup Greek yogurt (plain or vanilla)

1/2 cup unsweetened almond milk (or any milk of choice)

1-2 tablespoons sucralose (to taste)

1/2 teaspoon vanilla extract (optional)

Ice cubes (optional, for a thicker texture)

Instructions:

1. **Combine Ingredients:** In a blender, combine strawberries, flaxseeds, Greek yogurt, almond milk, sucralose, and vanilla extract (if using).
2. **Blend:** Blend until smooth and creamy.
3. **Adjust Thickness:** Add ice cubes if desired and blend again until the smoothie reaches your preferred thickness
4. **Taste and Adjust Sweetness:** Taste and adjust the sweetness by adding more sucralose if needed.
5. **Serve:** Pour into glasses and serve immediately for the best flavor and texture.

Nutrients (per serving)

Calories: 150 kcal Carbohydrates: 20g Fiber: 5g

Protein: 7g Fat: 5g Sugar: 8g Sodium: 60mg

Calcium: 200mg

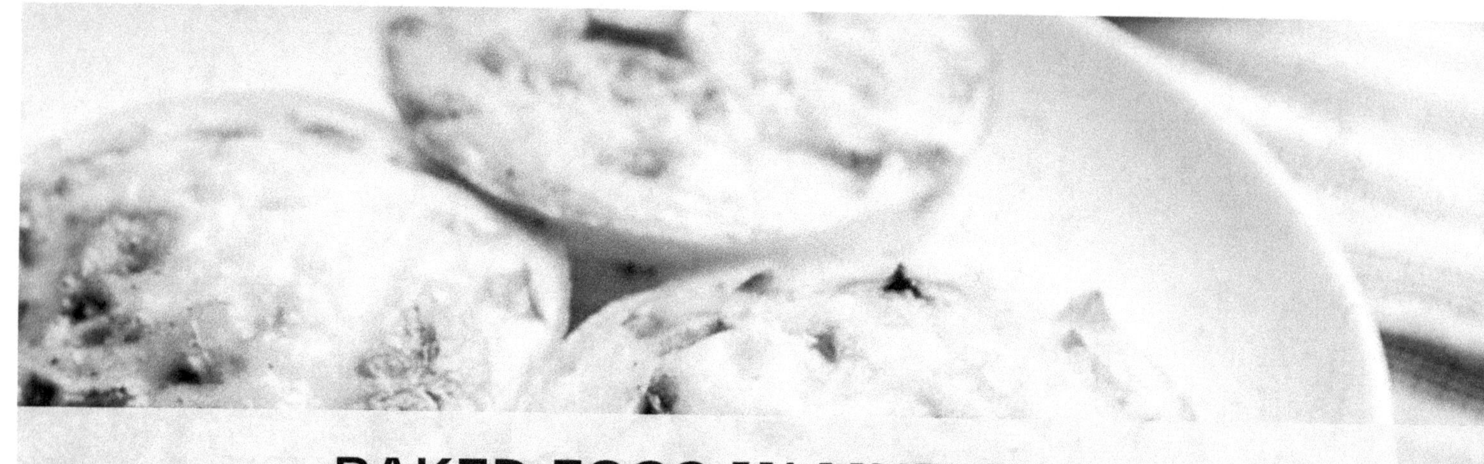

BAKED EGGS IN MUFFIN TIN

Baked Eggs in a Muffin Tin are a versatile and convenient breakfast option that can be customized to your taste. These protein-packed eggs are baked in a muffin tin, creating individual servings that are perfect for meal prep. They are seasoned with sucralose for a subtle touch of sweetness and combined with your favorite vegetables and proteins for a nutritious start to your day.

Serves		**Preparation Time**		**Cooking Time**	
4		10 minutes		20 minute	

Ingredients:

8 large eggs
1/4 cup milk (any type)
1/4 cup shredded cheese (optional)
1/2 cup diced bell peppers
1/2 cup chopped spinach
1/4 cup diced onions
1/2 teaspoon salt
1/4 teaspoon black pepper
1-2 tablespoons sucralose (to taste)
Cooking spray or olive oil for greasing the muffin tin

Instructions:

1. **Preheat the Oven:** Preheat the oven to 375°F (190°C). Grease a muffin tin with cooking spray or a light coating of olive oil.
2. **Mix Ingredients:** In a large bowl, whisk together the eggs, milk, sucralose, salt, and pepper until well combined. Stir in the shredded cheese (if using), diced bell peppers, chopped spinach, and diced onions.
3. **Pour Mixture:** Pour the egg mixture evenly into the prepared muffin tin cups, filling each about 3/4 full.
4. **Bake:** Bake in the preheated oven for 18-20 minutes, or until the eggs are fully set and the tops are slightly golden.
5. **Cool and Serve:** Remove from the oven and allow to cool slightly before serving. Use a spoon to gently remove the baked eggs from the muffin tin.

Nutrients (per serving)

Calories: 130 kcal Carbohydrates: 2g Fiber: 1g
Protein: 10g Fat: 9g Sugar: 1g Sodium: 300mg
Calcium: 150mg

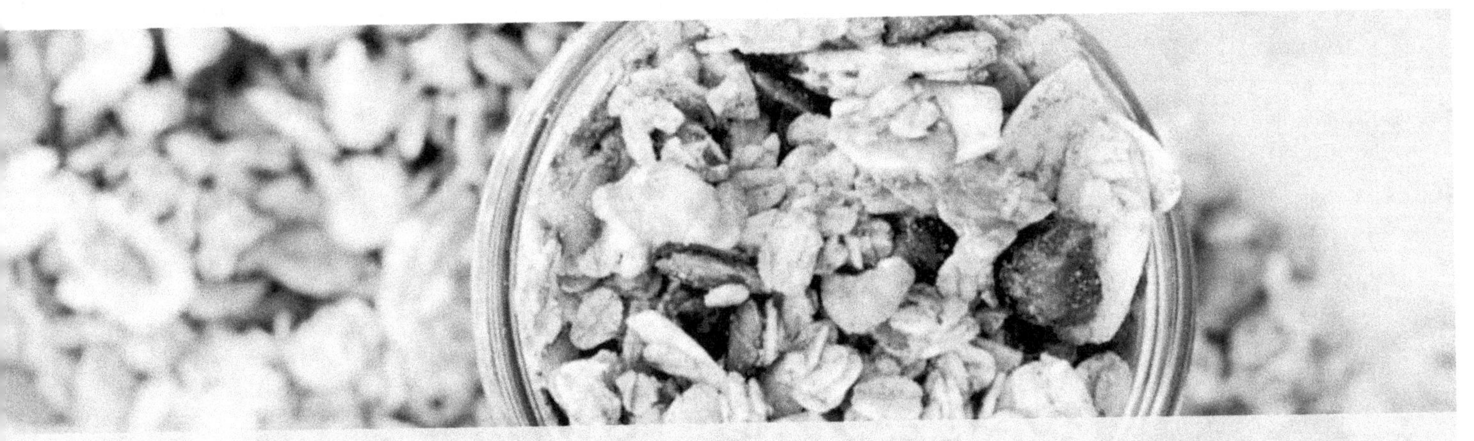

HOMEMADE SUGAR-FREE GRANOLA

Homemade Sugar-Free Granola is a crunchy, nutritious, and customizable snack or breakfast option that avoids added sugars. Sweetened with sucralose, this granola provides a satisfying crunch and natural sweetness without compromising your health goals. Packed with nuts, seeds, and a touch of dried fruit, it's perfect for topping yogurt, enjoying with milk, or eating straight from the jar.

Serves		**Preparation Time**		**Cooking Time**	
6		10 minutes		30 minute	

Ingredients:

2 cups old-fashioned rolled oats

1 cup chopped nuts (e.g., almonds, walnuts, pecans)

1/2 cup seeds (e.g., pumpkin seeds, sunflower seeds)

1/2 cup unsweetened shredded coconut

1/4 cup sucralose (adjust to taste)

1/2 teaspoon ground cinnamon

1/4 teaspoon salt

1/4 cup coconut oil or olive oil

1/4 cup pure vanilla extract

1/2 cup unsweetened dried fruit (e.g., raisins, cranberries, chopped apricots) (optional)

Instructions:

1. **Preheat the Oven:** Preheat the oven to 325°F (165°C). Line a baking sheet with parchment paper.
2. **Mix Dry Ingredients:** In a large bowl, combine the rolled oats, chopped nuts, seeds, shredded coconut, sucralose, ground cinnamon, and salt.
3. **Melt Oil and Vanilla:** In a small saucepan, heat the coconut oil and vanilla extract over low heat until melted and combined.
4. **Combine Mixtures:** Pour the melted oil and vanilla mixture over the dry ingredients and stir until everything is evenly coated.
5. **Bake:** Spread the mixture evenly on the prepared baking sheet. Bake in the preheated oven for 25-30 minutes, stirring once halfway through, until the granola is golden brown and crispy.
6. **Cool:** Remove from the oven and allow to cool completely on the baking sheet. It will become crispier as it cools.
7. **Add Dried Fruit (Optional):** Once cooled, stir in the dried fruit if using.

Nutrients (per serving)

Calories: 200 kcal Carbohydrates: 20g Fiber: 4g

Protein: 5g Fat: 12g Sugar: 2g Sodium: 100mg

Calcium: 50mg

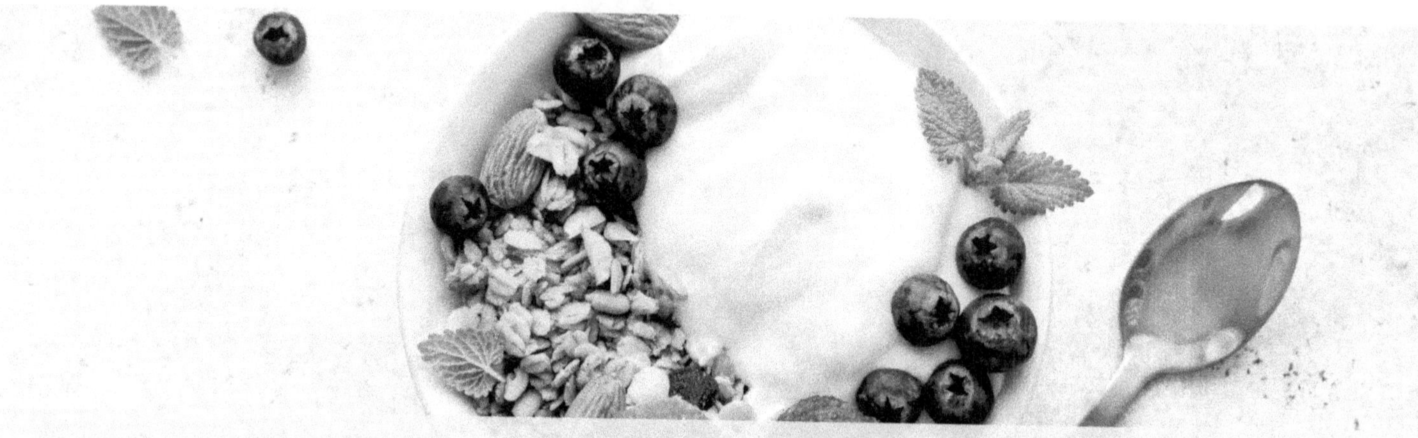

GREEK YOGURT WITH BERRIES AND CASHEWS

Greek Yogurt with Berries and Cashews is a refreshing and protein-packed breakfast or snack that's both satisfying and nutritious. The creamy texture of Greek yogurt paired with the natural sweetness of fresh berries and the crunch of cashews creates a perfect balance of flavors and textures. This recipe is quick to prepare and provides a wholesome, low-sugar option for any time of day.

Serves		**Preparation Time**		**Cooking Time**	
4		5 minutes		0 minute	

Ingredients:

2 cups plain Greek yogurt (non-fat or low-fat)
1 cup mixed fresh berries (e.g., strawberries, blueberries, raspberries)
1/4 cup cashews, chopped
1 tablespoon sucralose (adjust to taste)
1 teaspoon vanilla extract (optional)

Instructions:

1. **Prepare the Yogurt:** In a medium bowl, stir the Greek yogurt until smooth. If using vanilla extract, mix it into the yogurt.
2. **Add Sweetener:** Gently fold in the sucralose until evenly distributed. Taste and adjust sweetness if needed.
3. **Divide into Bowls:** Divide the yogurt among four serving bowls.
4. **Add Toppings:** Top each bowl with an equal amount of mixed fresh berries and chopped cashews.
5. **Serve:** Serve immediately or refrigerate until ready to eat.

Nutrients (per serving)

Calories: 180 kcal Carbohydrates: 15g Fiber: 3g
Protein: 15g Fat: 8g Sugar: 8g Sodium: 60mg
Calcium: 200mg

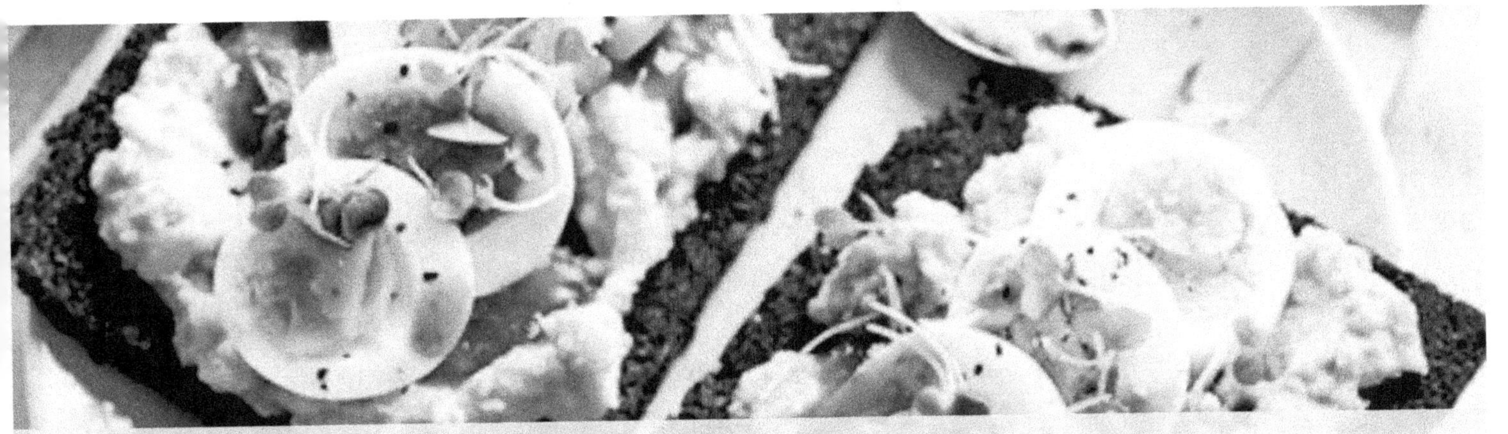

EGG AND AVOCADO SANDWICH

The Egg and Avocado Sandwich is a delicious and nutritious meal that combines creamy avocado with a protein-rich egg for a satisfying and balanced bite. This sandwich is perfect for breakfast or a quick lunch, offering a hearty dose of healthy fats, proteins, and essential nutrients. The simple ingredients come together to create a tasty and wholesome option that keeps you feeling full and energized.

Serves	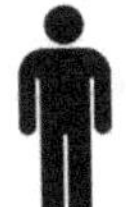	Preparation Time		Cooking Time	
4		10 minutes		10 minute	

Ingredients:

4 large eggs
1 ripe avocado, peeled and sliced
4 whole-grain sandwich bread slices
1 tablespoon olive oil or butter
Salt and pepper to taste
1 tablespoon sucralose (optional, for a slight touch of sweetness)
1 teaspoon lemon juice (optional, to prevent avocado browning)
Fresh herbs (e.g., parsley or chives) for garnish (optional)

Instructions:

1. **Cook the Eggs:** Heat olive oil or butter in a non-stick skillet over medium heat. Crack the eggs into the skillet and cook to your preferred doneness (sunny-side up, over-easy, or scrambled). Season with salt and pepper.
2. **Toast the Bread:** While the eggs are cooking, toast the whole-grain bread slices until golden brown.
3. **Prepare the Avocado:** If desired, mix the avocado slices with lemon juice and sucralose to enhance flavor and prevent browning.
4. **Assemble the Sandwich:** Once the bread is toasted, place the avocado slices on two of the bread slices, spreading them evenly. Top the avocado with the cooked eggs.
5. **Season and Garnish:** Season with additional salt and pepper if needed, and garnish with fresh herbs if desired. Top with the remaining bread slices to complete the sandwich.
6. **Serve:** Serve immediately.

Nutrients (per serving)

Calories: 290 kcal Carbohydrates: 22g Fiber: 7g

Protein: 15g Fat: 16g Sugar: 2g Sodium: 320mg

Calcium: 70mg

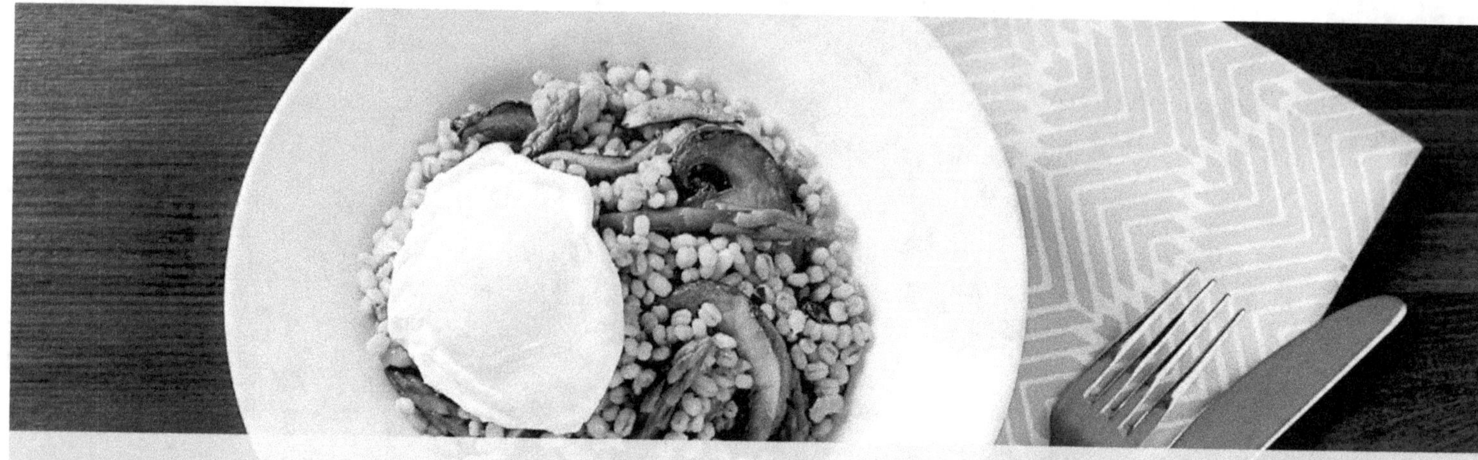

BARLEY PORRIDGE WITH MUSHROOMS AND POACHED EGG

Barley Porridge with Mushrooms and Poached Egg is a savory and hearty dish that blends the nutty flavors of barley with the umami richness of mushrooms and the creamy texture of a poached egg. This meal is ideal for breakfast or a light lunch, offering a well-rounded combination of whole grains, vegetables, and protein. It's a perfect option for those seeking a nutritious and comforting meal.

Serves	 **Preparation Time**		**Cooking Time**	
4	15 minutes		30 minute	

Ingredients:

1 cup pearl barley
4 cups low-sodium vegetable or chicken broth
1 tablespoon olive oil
1 medium onion, finely chopped
2 cloves garlic, minced
1 cup mushrooms, sliced (such as cremini or button)
1 teaspoon dried thyme
Salt and pepper to taste
4 large eggs
2 tablespoons white vinegar (for poaching eggs)
Fresh parsley, chopped (for garnish)

Instructions:

1. **Cook the Barley:** Rinse the barley under cold water. In a medium pot, bring the vegetable or chicken broth to a boil. Add the barley, reduce heat to low, cover, and simmer for about 25-30 minutes, or until the barley is tender and has absorbed most of the liquid. Stir occasionally.
2. **Sauté the Vegetables:** While the barley is cooking, heat olive oil in a large skillet over medium heat. Add the chopped onion and garlic, and sauté until softened, about 5 minutes.
3. **Cook the Mushrooms:** Add the sliced mushrooms and dried thyme to the skillet. Cook until the mushrooms are tender and browned, about 8-10 minutes. Season with salt and pepper.
4. **Poach the Eggs:** In a separate pot, bring water to a gentle simmer and add the white vinegar. Crack each egg into a small bowl and gently slide into the simmering water. Poach for 3-4 minutes, or until the whites are set and the yolks are still runny. Remove with a slotted spoon and set aside.
5. **Combine Barley and Mushroom Mixture:** Once the barley is cooked, stir in the mushroom mixture. Adjust seasoning with additional salt and pepper if needed.
6. **Serve:** Divide the barley porridge among four bowls. Top each bowl with a poached egg. Garnish with fresh parsley and serve immediately.

Nutrients (per serving)

Calories: 320 kcal Carbohydrates: 45g Fiber: 6g
Protein: 14g Fat: 9g Sugar: 2g Sodium: 410mg
Calcium: 30mg

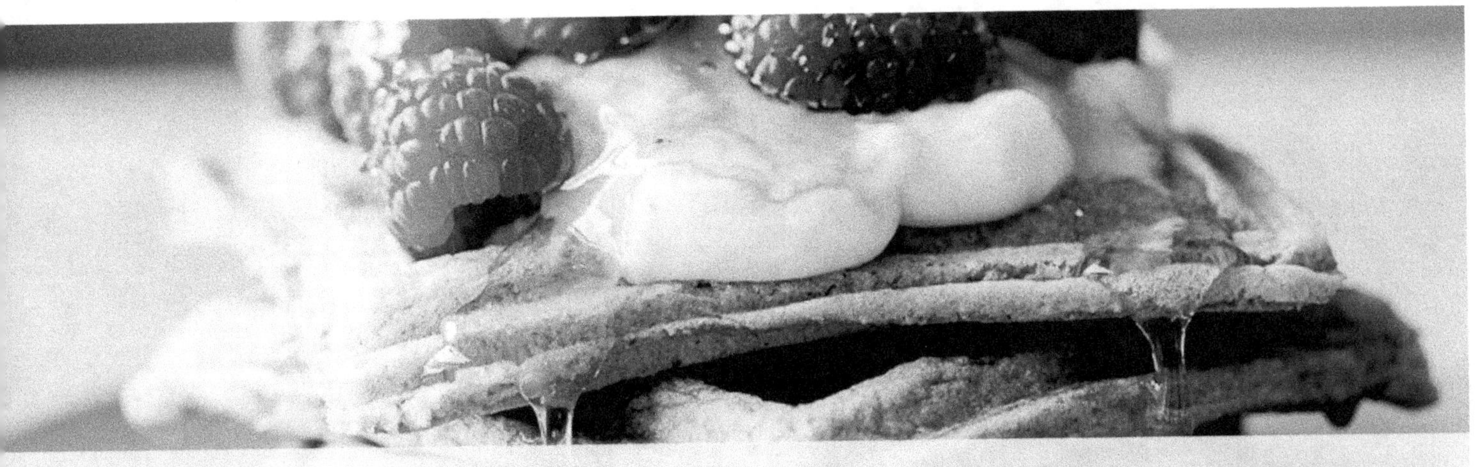

HEALTHY WAFFLES

Healthy Waffles offer a delightful, guilt-free breakfast option that combines wholesome ingredients for a nutritious start to your day. These waffles are light yet filling, incorporating whole grains and natural sweetness. Perfect for meal prepping, they can be enjoyed fresh or frozen for a quick and easy breakfast.

Serves		**Preparation Time**		**Cooking Time**	
4	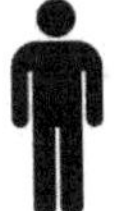	10 minutes		15 minute	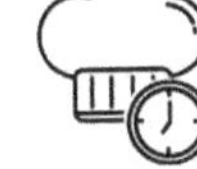

Ingredients:

1 cup whole wheat flour

1/2 cup oat flour

2 tablespoons sucralose

1 tablespoon baking powder

1/2 teaspoon salt

1 cup almond milk (or any milk of choice)

1/4 cup plain Greek yogurt

2 large eggs

2 tablespoons melted coconut oil

1 teaspoon vanilla extract

Instructions:

1. **Preheat the Waffle Iron:** Preheat your waffle iron according to the manufacturer's instructions.
2. **Prepare Dry Ingredients:** In a large bowl, whisk together the whole wheat flour, oat flour, sucralose, baking powder, and salt.
3. **Mix Wet Ingredients:** In another bowl, combine almond milk, Greek yogurt, eggs, melted coconut oil, and vanilla extract. Mix until well combined.
4. **Combine Ingredients:** Pour the wet ingredients into the dry ingredients and stir until just combined. Be careful not to overmix; lumps are okay.
5. **Cook the Waffles:** Lightly grease the waffle iron with cooking spray or additional melted coconut oil. Pour batter onto the preheated waffle iron (amount will depend on the size of your waffle iron). Close the lid and cook according to the manufacturer's instructions, typically about 4-5 minutes, until the waffles are golden brown and crisp.
6. **Serve:** Carefully remove the waffles and repeat with the remaining batter. Serve warm with your favorite toppings.

Nutrients (per serving)

Calories: 200 kcal Carbohydrates: 28g Fiber: 4g

Protein: 8g Fat: 6g Sugar: 2g Sodium: 220mg

Calcium: 150mg

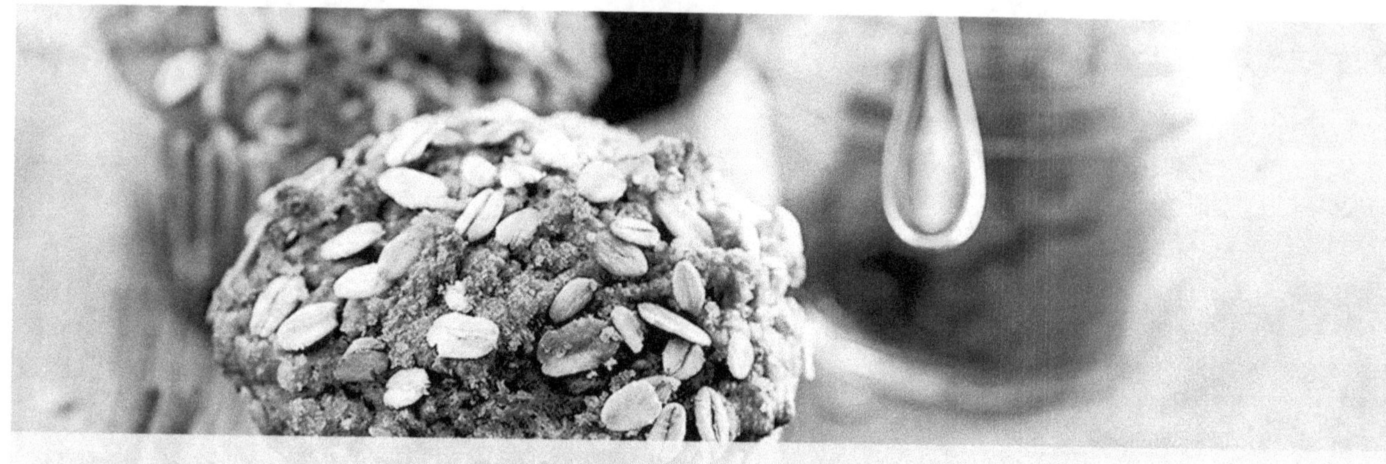

PUMPKIN OAT MUFFINS

Pumpkin Oat Muffins are a perfect blend of fall flavors and wholesome ingredients. These muffins are not only delicious but also packed with nutrients, making them an excellent choice for a healthy breakfast or snack. With the added benefit of sucralose for sweetness, these muffins offer a guilt-free indulgence.

Serves	**Preparation Time**	**Cooking Time**
12	10 minutes	20 minute

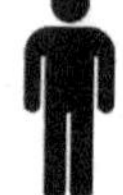
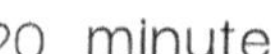

Ingredients:

1 cup rolled oats
1 cup whole wheat flour
1/2 cup canned pumpkin puree
1/4 cup sucralose
1/4 cup coconut oil, melted
1/2 cup almond milk (or any milk of choice)
2 large eggs
1 teaspoon baking powder
1/2 teaspoon baking soda
1/2 teaspoon ground cinnamon
1/4 teaspoon ground nutmeg
1/4 teaspoon salt
1/2 cup chopped walnuts (optional)

Instructions:

1. **Preheat the Oven:** Preheat your oven to 350°F (175°C) and line a muffin tin with paper liners or lightly grease it.
2. **Prepare Dry Ingredients:** In a medium bowl, combine the rolled oats, whole wheat flour, baking powder, baking soda, cinnamon, nutmeg, and salt.
3. **Mix Wet Ingredients:** In a separate large bowl, whisk together the pumpkin puree, sucralose, melted coconut oil, almond milk, and eggs until smooth and well combined.
4. **Combine Ingredients:** Gradually add the dry ingredients to the wet ingredients, mixing until just combined. Be careful not to overmix. Fold in the chopped walnuts if using.
5. **Bake the Muffins:** Divide the batter evenly among the muffin cups, filling each about 3/4 full. Bake for 20 minutes, or until a toothpick inserted into the center of a muffin comes out clean.
6. **Cool and Serve:** Allow the muffins to cool in the tin for 5 minutes before transferring them to a wire rack to cool completely.

Nutrients (per serving)

Calories: 150 kcal Carbohydrates: 22g Fiber: 3g
Protein: 4g Fat: 6g Sugar: 3g Sodium: 180mg
Calcium: 60mg

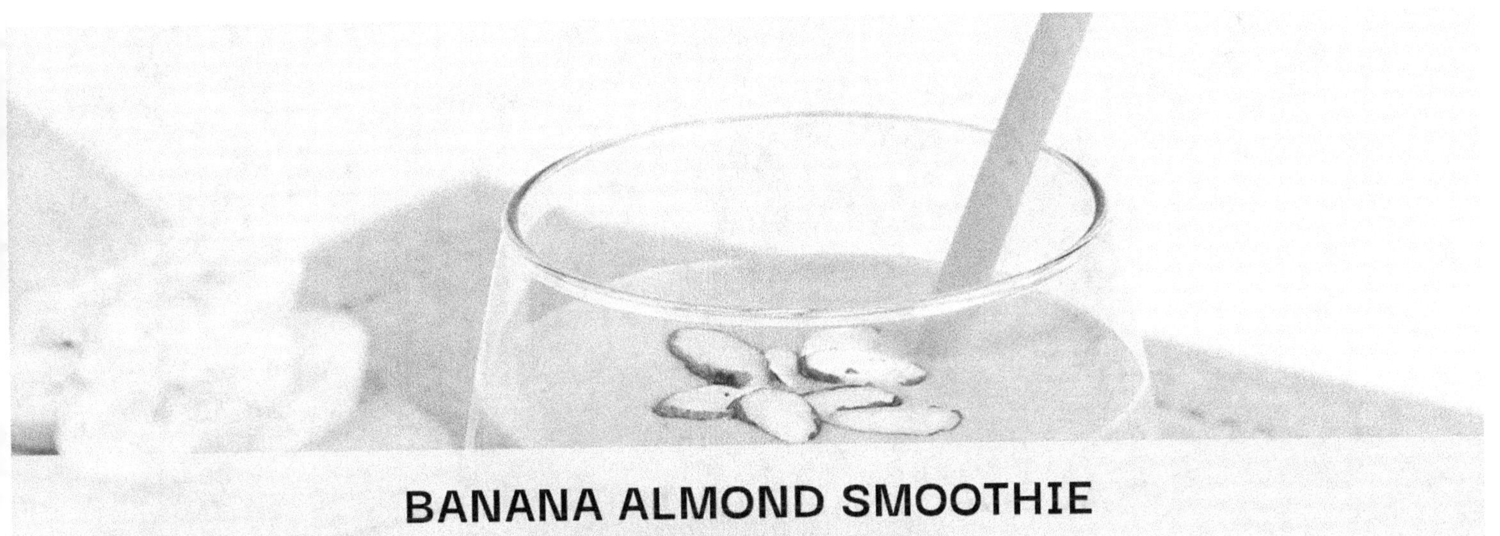

BANANA ALMOND SMOOTHIE

The Banana Almond Smoothie is a creamy, delicious, and nutritious drink that combines the natural sweetness of bananas with the rich flavor of almonds. This smoothie is perfect for a quick breakfast or a satisfying snack, offering a healthy dose of protein, fiber, and essential nutrients.

Serves		Preparation Time		Cooking Time	
2		5 minutes		0 minute	

Ingredients:

2 ripe bananas

1/4 cup almond butter

1 cup almond milk (or any milk of choice)

1 tablespoon sucralose

1/2 teaspoon vanilla extract

1/4 teaspoon ground cinnamon (optional)

Ice cubes (optional)

Instructions:

1. **Prepare Ingredients:** Peel the bananas and cut them into chunks.
2. **Blend the Smoothie:** In a blender, combine the banana chunks, almond butter, almond milk, sucralose, and vanilla extract.
3. **Adjust Consistency and Sweetness:** Blend until smooth and creamy. If you prefer a colder smoothie, add a few ice cubes and blend again until well combined.
4. **Taste and Final Adjustments:** Taste and adjust sweetness if needed by adding a bit more sucralose. Blend briefly to mix.
5. **Serve:** Pour the smoothie into glasses and serve immediately.

Nutrients (per serving)

Calories: 210 kcal Carbohydrates: 28g Fiber: 4g

Protein: 6g Fat: 9g Sugar: 14g Sodium: 80mg

Calcium: 300mg

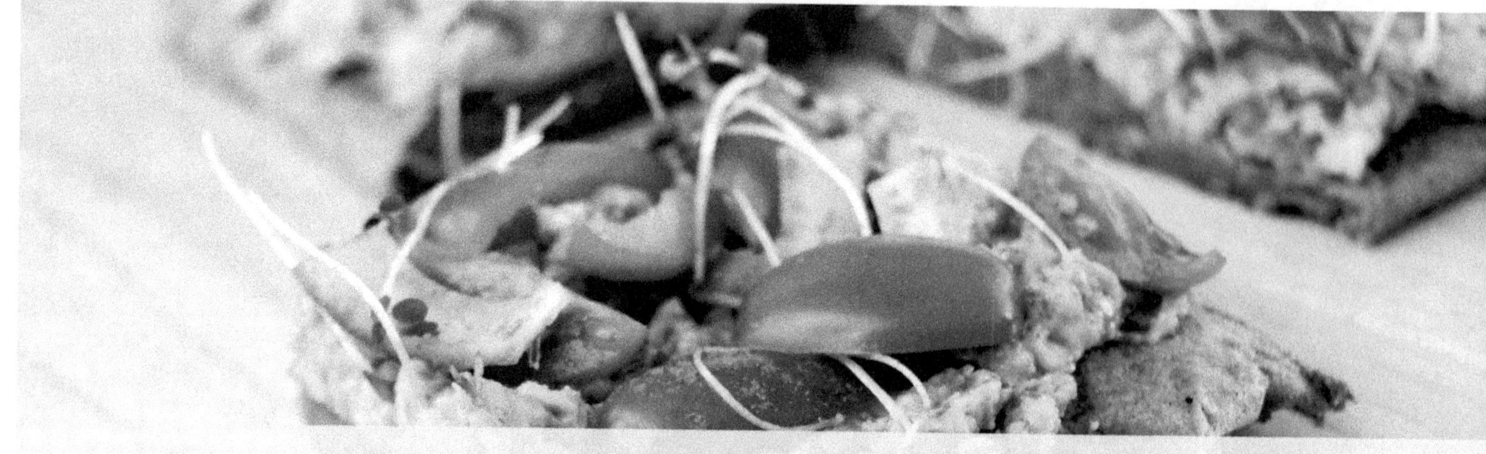

AVOCADO AND QUINOA TOAST

Avocado and Quinoa Toast is a wholesome, nutritious, and delicious meal that pairs creamy avocado with protein-packed quinoa on crispy whole grain toast. This recipe is not only easy to prepare but also packed with healthy fats, fiber, and essential nutrients, making it a perfect choice for a satisfying breakfast or a light lunch.

Serves		**Preparation Time**		**Cooking Time**	
2		10 minutes		15 minute	

Ingredients:

2 slices whole grain bread
1/2 cup cooked quinoa
1 ripe avocado
1 tablespoon sucralose
1 tablespoon lemon juice
Salt and pepper to taste
Red pepper flakes (optional)
Fresh herbs for garnish (optional, such as cilantro
or parsley)

Instructions:

1. **Toast the Bread:** Toast the whole grain bread slices until they are crispy and golden brown.
2. **Prepare the Avocado Spread:** While the bread is toasting, in a small bowl, mash the avocado with the lemon juice and sucralose until smooth. Season with salt and pepper to taste.
3. **Assemble the Toast:** Spread a generous layer of the mashed avocado mixture onto each slice of toasted bread.
4. **Add the Quinoa:** Top the avocado spread with cooked quinoa, spreading it evenly over the toast.
5. **Season and Serve:** Sprinkle with red pepper flakes and fresh herbs, if using. Serve immediately for the best texture and flavor.

Nutrients (per serving)

Calories: 320 kcal Carbohydrates: 40g Fiber: 8g

Protein: 10g Fat: 14g Sugar: 2g Sodium: 250mg

Calcium: 60mg

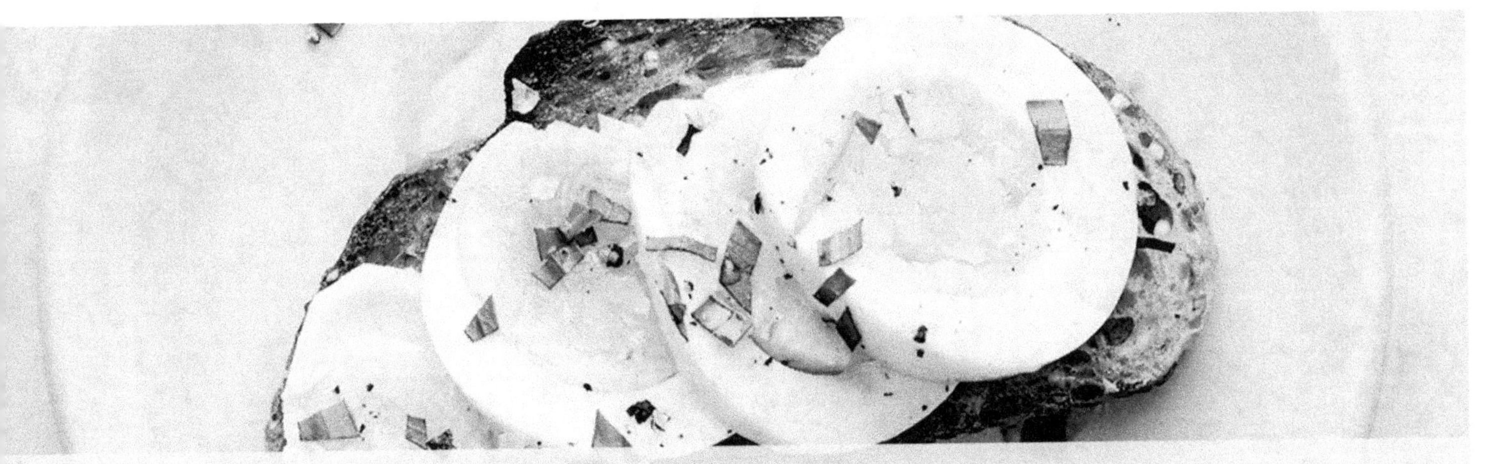

HARD-BOILED EGGS WITH WHOLE-GRAIN TOAST

Hard-Boiled Eggs with Whole-Grain Toast is a classic, nutritious meal that's both simple and satisfying. This recipe combines protein-rich hard-boiled eggs with fiber-packed whole-grain toast, making it a perfect choice for a balanced breakfast or a quick, healthy lunch. The addition of a touch of sucralose in the seasoning adds a subtle sweetness that complements the savory flavors.

Serves		Preparation Time		Cooking Time	
2		10 minutes		10 minute	

Ingredients:

4 large eggs
2 slices whole-grain bread
1 teaspoon sucralose
1 tablespoon olive oil
Salt and pepper to taste
Fresh chives or parsley for garnish (optional)

Instructions:

1. **Cook the Eggs:** Place the eggs in a saucepan and cover with cold water. Bring to a boil over medium-high heat.Once the water reaches a rolling boil, cover the saucepan with a lid and remove from heat. Let the eggs sit in the hot water for 10 minutes.After 10 minutes, transfer the eggs to a bowl of ice water to cool. Peel the eggs once they are cool enough to handle.
2. **Toast the Bread:** While the eggs are cooling, toast the whole-grain bread slices until they are crispy and golden brown.
3. **Prepare the Eggs:** Slice the peeled hard-boiled eggs and season with sucralose, salt, and pepper to taste.
4. **Assemble the Toast:** Drizzle olive oil over the toasted bread slices and top with the sliced eggs.
5. **Garnish and Serve:** Garnish with fresh chives or parsley if desired. Serve immediately.

Nutrients (per serving)

Calories: 290 kcal Carbohydrates: 28g Fiber: 6g
Protein: 15g Fat: 14g Sugar: 2g Sodium: 280mg
Calcium: 60mg

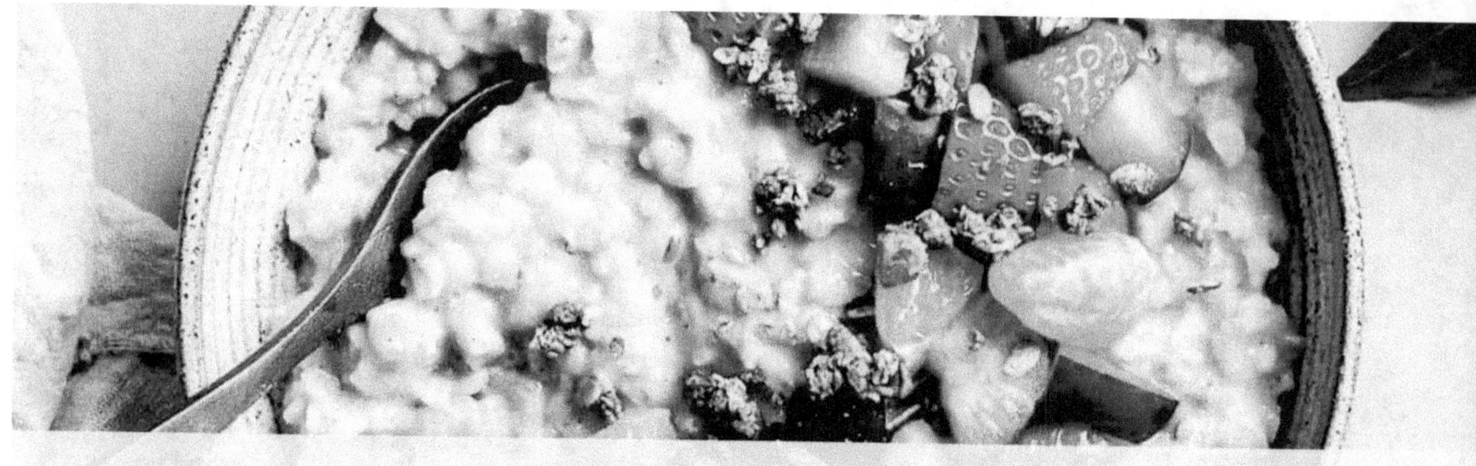

OATMEAL WITH WALNUTS AND HONEY

Oatmeal with Walnuts and Honey is a comforting and nutritious breakfast option that combines the heartiness of oats with the rich flavors of toasted walnuts and a drizzle of honey. This recipe provides a perfect balance of fiber, protein, and healthy fats, making it an ideal start to your day. The addition of sucralose helps to enhance the sweetness naturally without adding extra sugar.

Serves		Preparation Time		Cooking Time	
2		5 minutes		10 minute	

Ingredients:

1 cup rolled oats
2 cups water or low-fat milk
1/4 cup walnuts, chopped
2 tablespoons honey
1 teaspoon sucralose
1/2 teaspoon ground cinnamon
A pinch of salt

Instructions:

1. **Cook the Oats:** In a medium saucepan, bring the water or milk to a boil over medium-high heat.Add the rolled oats and a pinch of salt. Reduce the heat to low and simmer for about 5 minutes, stirring occasionally, until the oats are soft and have absorbed most of the liquid.
2. **Toast the Walnuts:** While the oats are cooking, toast the chopped walnuts in a small skillet over medium heat for 2-3 minutes, until they are fragrant and lightly browned. Stir frequently to prevent burning.
3. **Finish the Oatmeal:** Once the oats are cooked, stir in the sucralose and ground cinnamon.
4. **Assemble and Serve:** Divide the oatmeal between two bowls. Drizzle each bowl with honey and sprinkle with the toasted walnuts.
5. **Enjoy:** Serve warm and enjoy your delicious breakfast!

Nutrients (per serving)

Calories: 320 kcal Carbohydrates: 40g Fiber: 5g
Protein: 8g Fat: 14g Sugar: 12g Sodium: 150mg
Calcium: 90mg

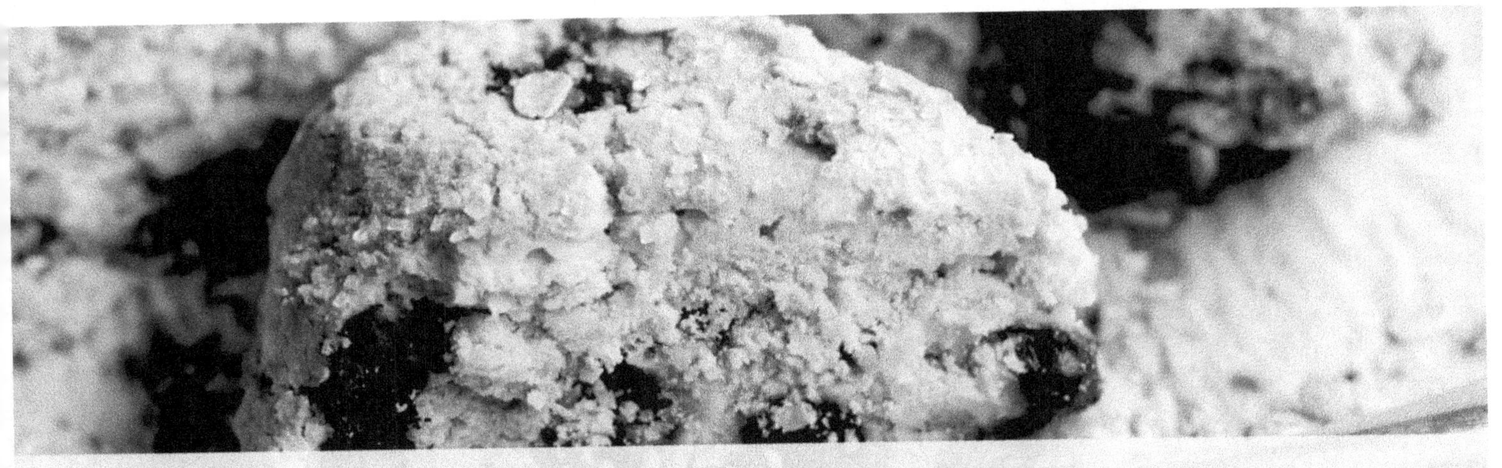

GLUTEN-FREE OAT SCONES

Gluten-Free Oat Scones are a delicious and wholesome treat perfect for breakfast or as a light snack. Made with gluten-free oats and sweetened with a touch of sucralose, these scones are soft, slightly crumbly, and packed with flavor. They offer a satisfying bite while being gentle on your digestive system.

Serves		Preparation Time		Cooking Time	
8	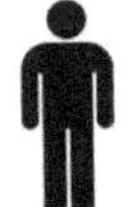	10 minutes		20 minute	

Ingredients:

1 1/2 cups gluten-free oat flour

1/2 cup gluten-free rolled oats

1/4 cup sucralose

1/2 cup unsalted butter, cold and cut into small pieces

1/2 teaspoon baking powder

1/4 teaspoon baking soda

1/4 teaspoon salt

1/2 cup milk (dairy or non-dairy)

1 large egg

1/2 teaspoon vanilla extract

1/2 cup raisins or dried cranberries (optional)

Instructions:

1. **Preheat Oven and Prepare Baking Sheet:** Preheat your oven to 375°F (190°C) and line a baking sheet with parchment paper.
2. **Prepare Dry Ingredients:** In a large bowl, whisk together the gluten-free oat flour, gluten-free rolled oats, sucralose, baking powder, baking soda, and salt.
3. **Cut in the Butter:** Add the cold butter pieces to the dry ingredients. Using a pastry cutter or your fingers, cut the butter into the mixture until it resembles coarse crumbs.
4. **Mix Wet Ingredients:** In a separate bowl, whisk together the milk, egg, and vanilla extract.
5. **Combine Ingredients:** Pour the wet ingredients into the dry mixture and stir until just combined. If using, fold in the raisins or dried cranberries.
6. **Shape and Cut the Dough:** Turn the dough out onto a lightly floured surface and gently knead it a few times to bring it together. Pat the dough into a 1-inch thick circle and cut it into 8 wedges.
7. **Bake the Scones:** Place the wedges onto the prepared baking sheet. Bake for 18-20 minutes, or until the scones are golden brown and a toothpick inserted into the center comes out clean.
8. **Cool and Serve:** Let the scones cool on a wire rack before serving.

Nutrients (per serving)

Calories: 180 kcal Carbohydrates: 22g Fiber: 2g

Protein: 3g Fat: 8g Sugar: 5g Sodium: 150mg

Calcium: 50mg

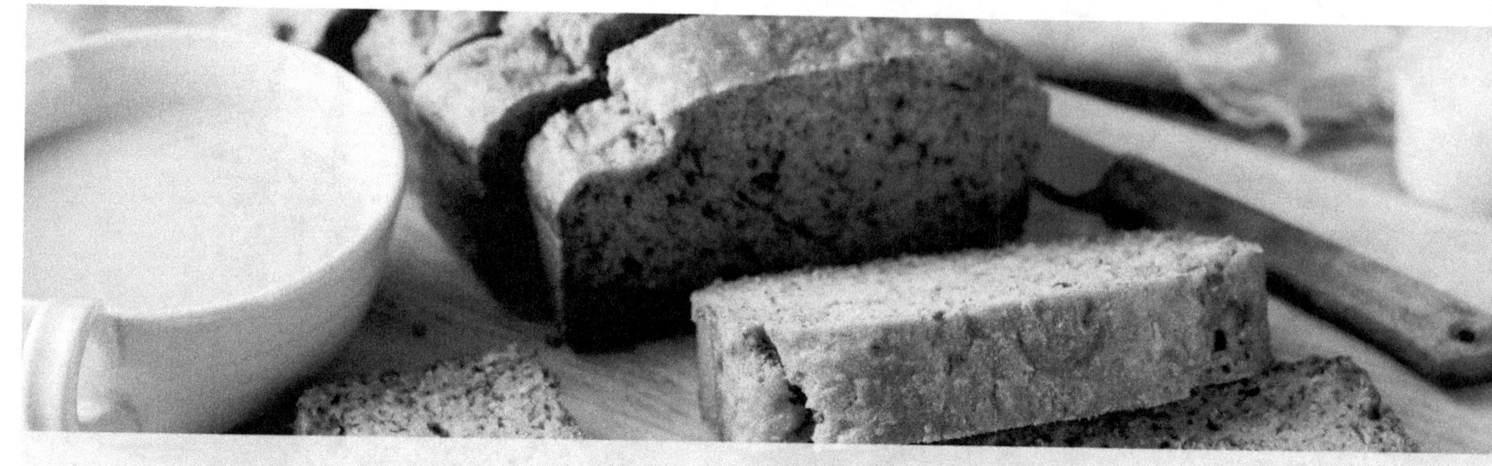

SUGAR-FREE BANANA BREAD

Sugar-Free Banana Bread is a delicious, moist, and naturally sweetened bread that's perfect for breakfast or as a snack. Using sucralose instead of sugar, this recipe offers a healthier option without sacrificing flavor. The ripe bananas provide natural sweetness, while the sucralose adds an extra touch of sweetness without the added calories.

Serves		**Preparation Time**		**Cooking Time**	
8		15 minutes		60 minute	

Ingredients:

2 to 3 ripe bananas, mashed (about 1 cup)
1/4 cup unsalted butter, softened
1/4 cup sucralose
2 large eggs
1 teaspoon vanilla extract
1 1/2 cups whole wheat flour
1 teaspoon baking powder
1/2 teaspoon baking soda
1/4 teaspoon salt
1/2 teaspoon ground cinnamon (optional)
1/2 cup chopped walnuts or pecans (optional)

Instructions:

1. **Preheat Oven and Prepare Pan:** Preheat your oven to 350°F (175°C). Grease and flour a 9x5-inch loaf pan or line it with parchment paper.
2. **Cream Butter and Sucralose:** In a large bowl, cream together the softened butter and sucralose until light and fluffy.
3. **Combine Wet Ingredients:** Add the mashed bananas, eggs, and vanilla extract to the butter mixture and mix until well combined.
4. **Prepare Dry Ingredients:** In a separate bowl, whisk together the whole wheat flour, baking powder, baking soda, salt, and ground cinnamon (if using).
5. **Combine Wet and Dry Ingredients:** Gradually add the dry ingredients to the wet ingredients, mixing just until combined. Be careful not to overmix.
6. **Fold in Nuts (if using):**
7. Fold in the chopped walnuts or pecans if using.
8. **Bake the Bread:** Pour the batter into the prepared loaf pan and smooth the top with a spatula. Bake for 55-60 minutes, or until a toothpick inserted into the center comes out clean.
9. **Cool and Slice:** Allow the bread to cool in the pan for 10 minutes, then transfer to a wire rack to cool completely before slicing.

Nutrients (per serving)

Calories: 180 kcal Carbohydrates: 25g Fiber: 3g
Protein: 4g Fat: 7g Sugar: 6g Sodium: 150mg
Calcium: 40mg

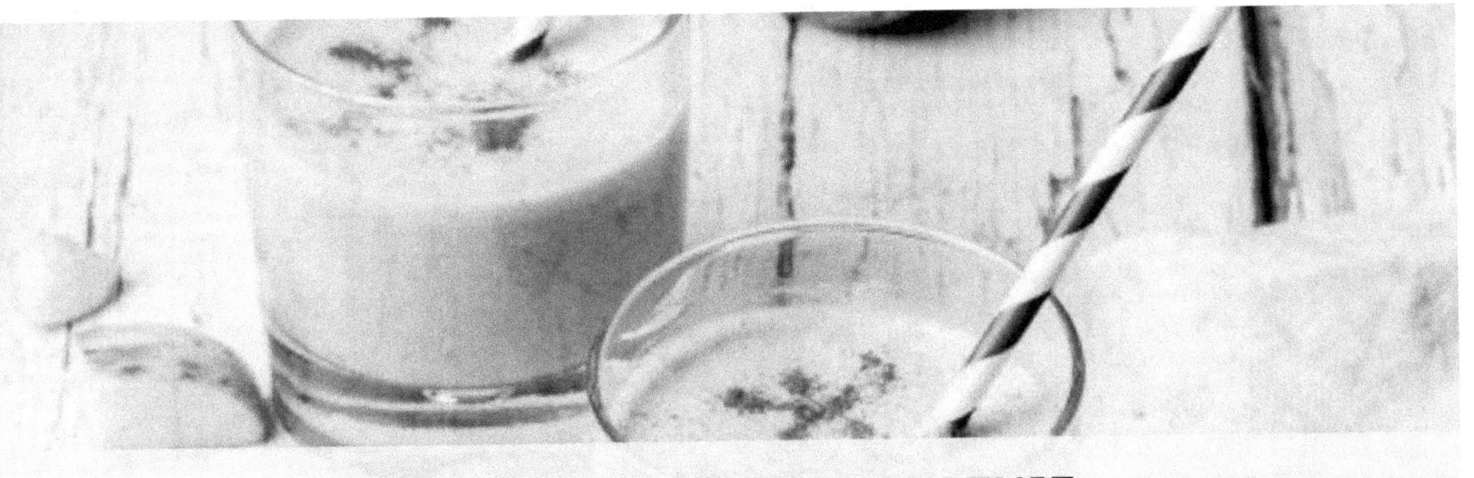

APPLE CINNAMON SMOOTHIE

The Apple Cinnamon Smoothie is a delicious and refreshing drink that combines the crisp taste of apples with the warm spice of cinnamon. It's perfect for a nutritious breakfast or a satisfying snack. Sweetened with sucralose, this smoothie offers a healthier alternative while still delivering a delightful taste.

Serves		Preparation Time		Cooking Time	
2		5 minutes		60 minute	

Ingredients:

1 large apple, peeled, cored, and chopped

1/2 cup Greek yogurt (plain or vanilla)

1/2 cup unsweetened almond milk (or any milk of your choice)

1 tablespoon sucralose

1/2 teaspoon ground cinnamon

1/2 teaspoon vanilla extract (optional)

1/2 cup ice cubes

Instructions:

1. **Prepare Ingredients:** Place the chopped apple, Greek yogurt, almond milk, sucralose, ground cinnamon, and vanilla extract (if using) into a blender.
2. **Blend:** Blend on high until smooth and creamy. Add ice cubes and blend again until the smoothie is chilled and frothy.
3. **Taste and Adjust:** Taste and adjust sweetness or cinnamon if needed.
4. **Serve:** Pour into glasses and serve immediately.

Nutrients (per serving)

Calories: 130 kcal Carbohydrates: 23g Fiber: 3g

Protein: 7g Fat: 2g Sugar: 11g Sodium: 60mg

Calcium: 150mg

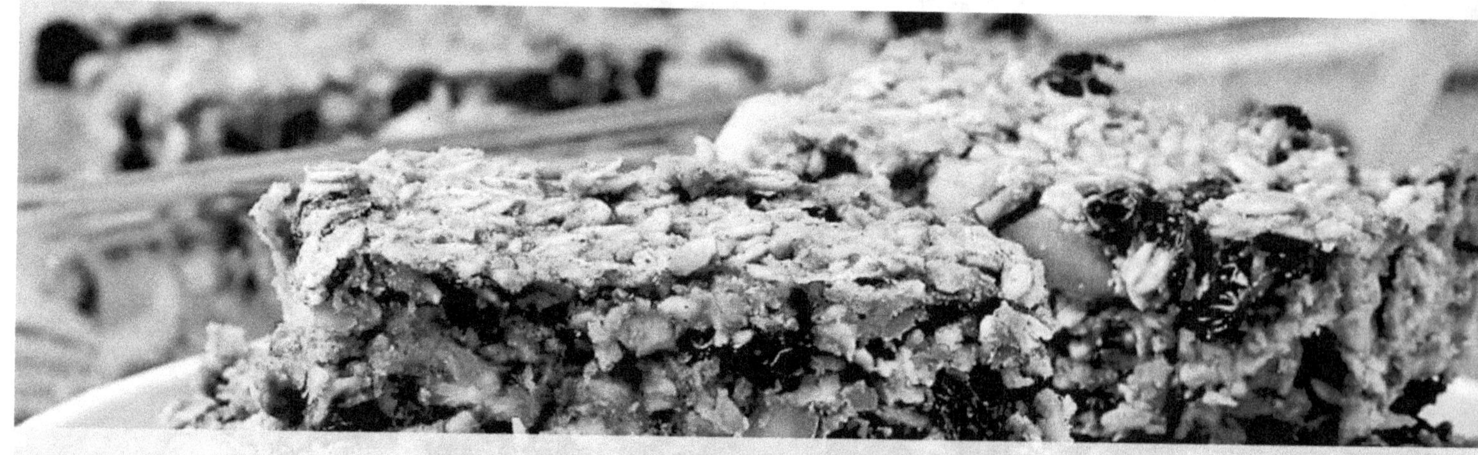

OATMEAL RAISIN BREAKFAST BARS

Oatmeal Raisin Breakfast Bars are a convenient and nutritious option for busy mornings or an afternoon pick-me-up. Made with wholesome ingredients and sweetened with sucralose, these bars offer a satisfying blend of oats, raisins, and a hint of cinnamon. They're perfect for meal prep and can be enjoyed on the go.

Serves	**Preparation Time**	**Cooking Time**
8	15 minutes	25 minute

  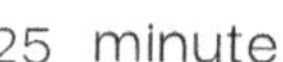

Ingredients:

- 2 cups old-fashioned oats
- 1/2 cup whole wheat flour
- 1/2 teaspoon baking powder
- 1/2 teaspoon ground cinnamon
- 1/4 teaspoon salt
- 1/4 cup unsalted butter, melted
- 1/4 cup sucralose
- 1/4 cup honey or maple syrup
- 1 large egg
- 1/2 cup raisins
- 1/4 cup chopped walnuts (optional)

Instructions:

1. **Preheat Oven:** Preheat your oven to 350°F (175°C) and line an 8x8-inch baking pan with parchment paper.
2. **Combine Dry Ingredients:** In a large bowl, combine the oats, whole wheat flour, baking powder, ground cinnamon, and salt.
3. **Mix Wet Ingredients:** In a separate bowl, whisk together the melted butter, sucralose, honey (or maple syrup), and egg until well combined.
4. **Combine Mixtures:** Pour the wet ingredients into the dry ingredients and mix until just combined. Stir in the raisins and walnuts if using.
5. **Prepare for Baking:** Spread the mixture evenly in the prepared baking pan and press it down firmly.
6. **Bake:** Bake for 25 minutes, or until the edges are golden brown and a toothpick inserted into the center comes out clean.
7. **Cool and Slice:** Allow the bars to cool in the pan for 10 minutes before transferring them to a wire rack to cool completely. Once cooled, cut into 8 bars.
8. **Store:** Store in an airtight container.

Nutrients (per serving)

Calories: 160 kcal Carbohydrates: 23g Fiber: 3g

Protein: 3g Fat: 6g Sugar: 10g Sodium: 100mg

Calcium: 30mg

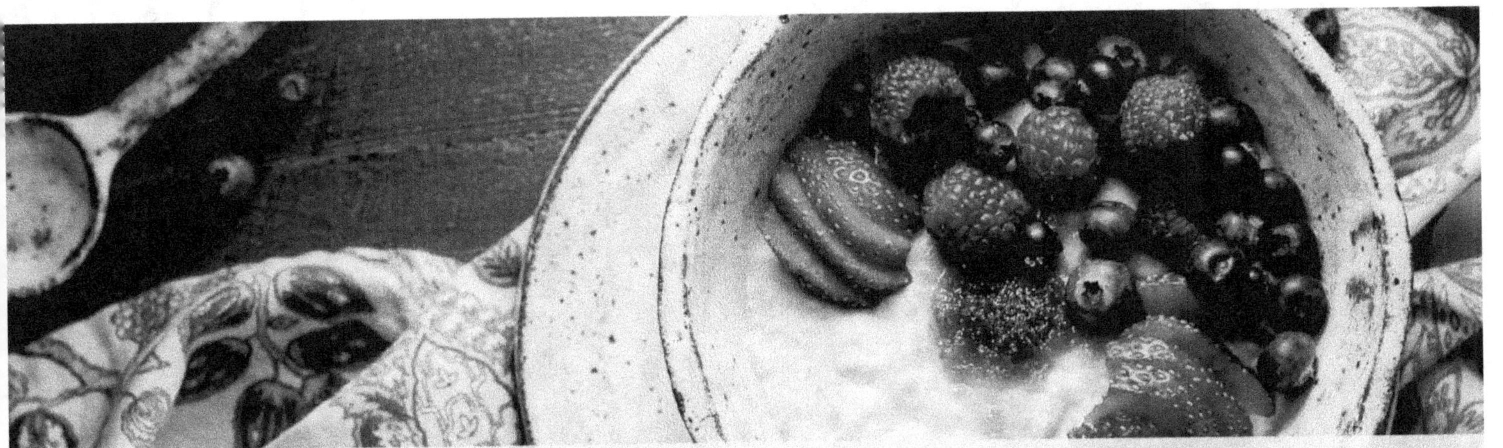

ALMOND FLOUR PORRIDGE WITH STRAWBERRIES

Almond Flour Porridge with Strawberries is a delicious and low-carb alternative to traditional oatmeal. This creamy and satisfying breakfast combines almond flour with fresh strawberries, providing a delightful start to your day. It's perfect for those following a low-carb or gluten-free diet and can be easily prepared ahead of time for a quick and nutritious breakfast.

Serves	Preparation Time	Cooking Time
2 	5 minutes 	10 minute 

Ingredients:

- 1 cup almond flour
- 1 cup unsweetened almond milk
- 1 tablespoon sucralose
- 1/2 teaspoon vanilla extract
- 1/2 teaspoon ground cinnamon
- 1/2 cup fresh strawberries, chopped
- 1 tablespoon chopped almonds (optional)

Instructions:

1. **Combine Ingredients:** In a medium saucepan, combine the almond flour, almond milk, sucralose, vanilla extract, and ground cinnamon.
2. **Cook Porridge:** Heat the mixture over medium heat, stirring continuously, until it begins to thicken and bubble, about 5-7 minutes.
3. **Simmer:** Reduce the heat to low and continue cooking for an additional 2-3 minutes, stirring frequently, until the porridge reaches your desired consistency.
4. **Finish and Serve:** Remove from heat and let it sit for a minute to cool slightly. Stir in the chopped strawberries and top with chopped almonds if desired.
5. **Enjoy:** Serve warm.

Nutrients (per serving)

Calories: 220 kcal Carbohydrates: 14g Fiber: 5g

Protein: 7g Fat: 15g Sugar: 5g Sodium: 200mg

Calcium: 300mg

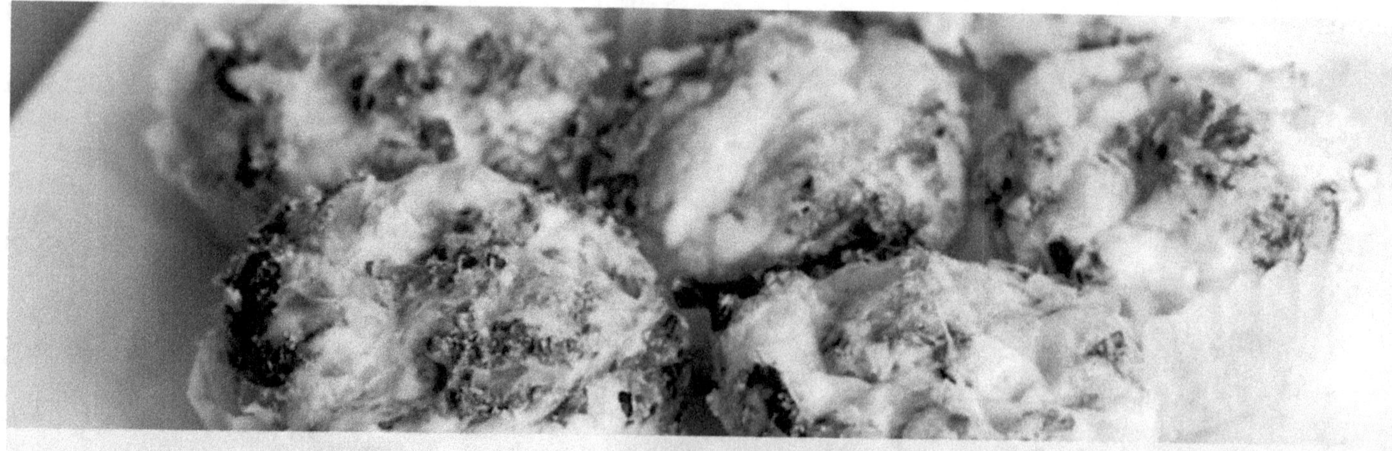

KALE AND CHEESE BAKED EGG CUPS

Kale and Cheese Baked Egg Cups are a perfect breakfast or snack option that's both nutritious and easy to prepare. These egg cups are packed with leafy kale, savory cheese, and eggs, providing a hearty start to your day. Baked to perfection, they are great for meal prep and can be enjoyed warm or cold.

Serves	 **Preparation Time**	**Cooking Time**	
4	10 minutes	20 minute	

Ingredients:

1 cup kale, finely chopped
1/2 cup shredded cheddar cheese
4 large eggs
1/4 cup milk (any kind)
1 tablespoon sucralose
1/2 teaspoon garlic powder
1/4 teaspoon salt
1/4 teaspoon black pepper
Cooking spray or a small amount of oil for greasing

Instructions:

1. **Preheat Oven:** Preheat your oven to 375°F (190°C). Lightly grease a muffin tin with cooking spray or a small amount of oil.
2. **Prepare Mixture:** In a medium bowl, combine the chopped kale, shredded cheddar cheese, sucralose, garlic powder, salt, and black pepper.
3. **Fill Muffin Tin:** Divide the kale and cheese mixture evenly among the muffin tin cups.
4. **Prepare Egg Mixture:** In a separate bowl, whisk together the eggs and milk until well combined.
5. **Assemble and Bake:** Pour the egg mixture over the kale and cheese mixture in each muffin cup, filling each about three-quarters full. Bake in the preheated oven for 20 minutes, or until the eggs are set and the tops are lightly golden.
6. **Cool and Serve:** Allow the egg cups to cool slightly before removing them from the muffin tin. Serve warm or store in the refrigerator for up to 5 days.

Nutrients (per serving)

Calories: 150 kcal Carbohydrates: 4g Fiber: 1g
Protein: 10g Fat: 10g Sugar: 1g Sodium: 290mg
Calcium: 150mg

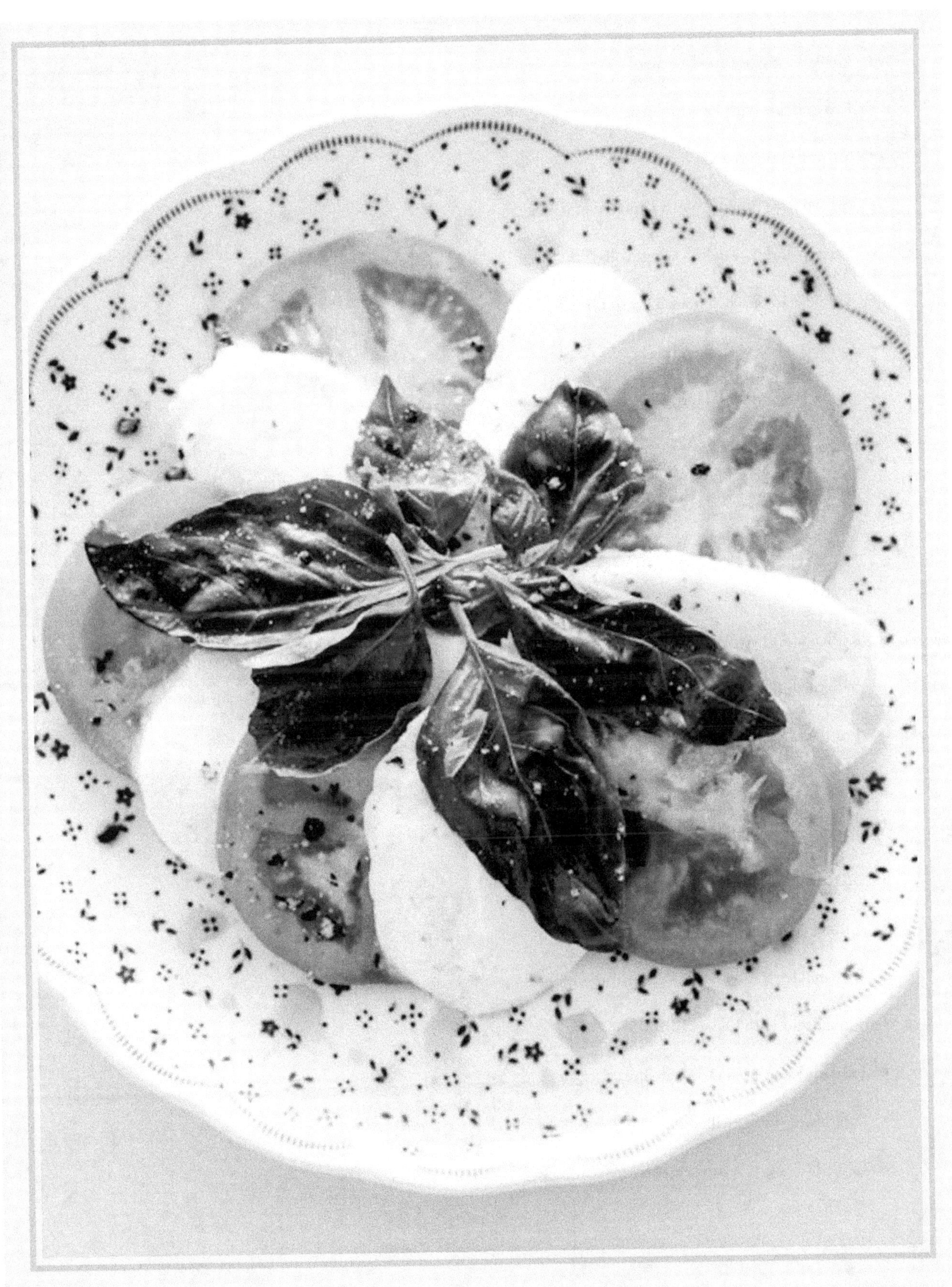

TABLE OF CONTENTS

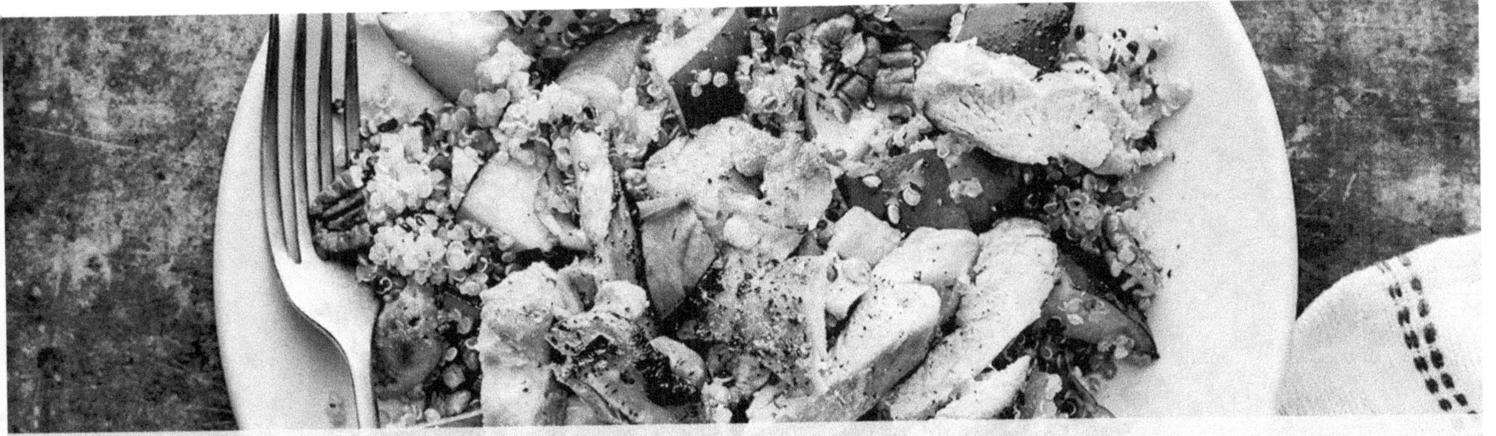

GRILLED CHICKEN AND QUINOA SALAD

Grilled Chicken and Quinoa Salad is a refreshing and satisfying dish that combines the lean protein of grilled chicken with the nutty flavor of quinoa and fresh, crisp vegetables. This salad is perfect for a healthy lunch or dinner, offering a balanced meal that is rich in nutrients and flavor. It's also great for meal prepping, as it stays fresh in the refrigerator for several days.

Serves		Preparation Time		Cooking Time	
4		15 minutes		20 minute	

Ingredients:

- 2 boneless, skinless chicken breasts
- 1 cup quinoa, rinsed
- 2 cups water or low-sodium chicken broth
- 1 red bell pepper, diced
- 1 cucumber, diced
- 1/2 red onion, finely chopped
- 1 cup cherry tomatoes, halved
- 1/4 cup fresh parsley, chopped
- 1/4 cup crumbled feta cheese (optional)
- 2 tablespoons olive oil
- 2 tablespoons lemon juice
- 1 tablespoon sucralose
- 1 teaspoon dried oregano
- 1/2 teaspoon garlic powder
- Salt and pepper to taste

Instructions:

1. **Preheat Grill:** Preheat the grill to medium-high heat.
2. **Season and Grill Chicken:** Season the chicken breasts with salt, pepper, and dried oregano. Grill the chicken for 6-7 minutes per side, or until fully cooked and the internal temperature reaches 165°F (74°C). Remove from the grill and let rest for 5 minutes before slicing.
3. **Cook Quinoa:** In a medium saucepan, bring the water or chicken broth to a boil. Add the quinoa, reduce heat to low, cover, and simmer for 15 minutes, or until the quinoa is tender and the liquid is absorbed. Fluff with a fork and let cool.
4. **Prepare Salad:** In a large bowl, combine the cooked quinoa, diced red bell pepper, cucumber, red onion, cherry tomatoes, and chopped parsley.
5. **Make Dressing:** In a small bowl, whisk together the olive oil, lemon juice, sucralose, garlic powder, salt, and pepper.
6. **Assemble Salad:** Slice the grilled chicken and add it to the quinoa mixture.
7. Pour the dressing over the salad and toss to combine.
8. **Serve:** Sprinkle with crumbled feta cheese if desired. Serve immediately or refrigerate for up to 3 days.

Nutrients (per serving)

Calories: 320 kcal Carbohydrates: 30g Fiber: 4g

Protein: 30g Fat: 10g Sugar: 3g Sodium: 300mg

Calcium: 80mg

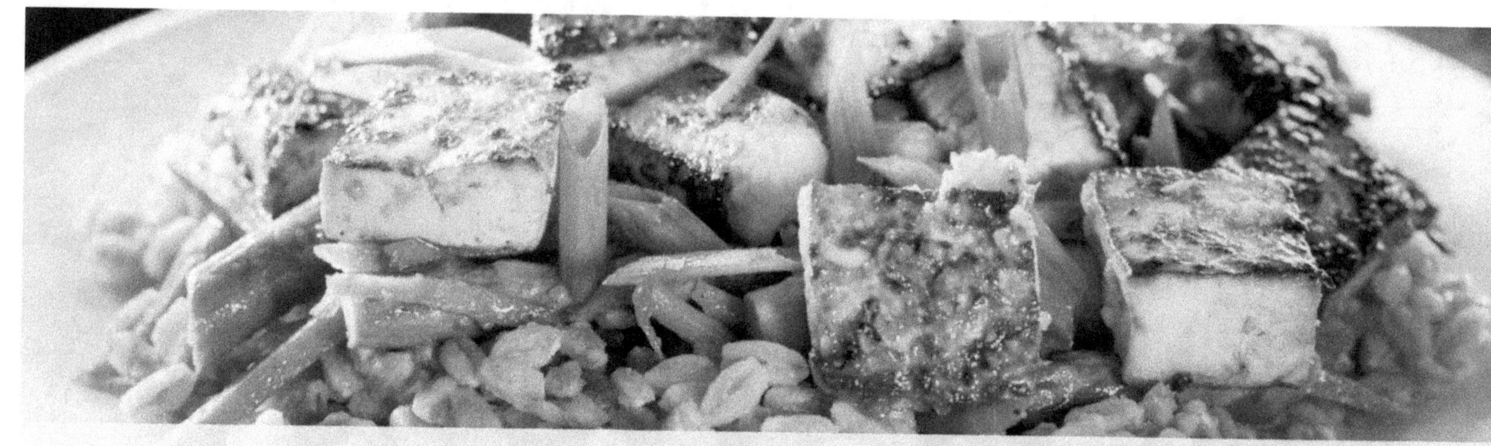

BROWN RICE WITH PEAS AND TOFU

Brown Rice with Peas and Tofu is a nourishing and flavorful dish that combines the wholesome goodness of brown rice with protein-packed tofu and sweet green peas. This vegetarian meal is perfect for a quick and healthy lunch or dinner, offering a balanced blend of carbohydrates, protein, and vegetables. It's a great option for meal prepping as it maintains its flavor and texture well in the refrigerator.

Serves		**Preparation Time**		**Cooking Time**	
4		10 minutes		25 minute	

Ingredients:

1 cup brown rice
2 cups water or vegetable broth
1 cup frozen peas
1 block (14 oz) firm tofu, drained and cubed
2 tablespoons olive oil
2 tablespoons soy sauce
1 tablespoon sucralose
2 cloves garlic, minced
1 teaspoon ginger, minced
1/2 teaspoon turmeric powder
1/2 teaspoon cumin powder
Salt and pepper to taste
2 green onions, chopped (for garnish)

Instructions:

1. **Cook Brown Rice:** Rinse the brown rice under cold water. In a medium saucepan, bring 2 cups of water or vegetable broth to a boil. Add the brown rice, reduce heat to low, cover, and simmer for 20-25 minutes, or until the rice is tender and the liquid is absorbed. Fluff with a fork and set aside.

2. **Cook Tofu:** While the rice is cooking, heat olive oil in a large skillet or wok over medium-high heat. Add the cubed tofu and cook for 5-7 minutes, turning occasionally, until golden brown on all sides. Remove the tofu from the skillet and set aside.

3. **Prepare Vegetables and Seasoning:** In the same skillet, add the minced garlic and ginger, cooking for 1 minute until fragrant.Add the frozen peas to the skillet and cook for 3-4 minutes, or until heated through.

4. **Combine Ingredients:** Stir in the turmeric powder, cumin powder, soy sauce, sucralose, salt, and pepper. Mix well.Return the tofu to the skillet and toss to combine with the peas and seasoning.

5. **Finish the Dish:** Add the cooked brown rice to the skillet and stir to combine all the ingredients. Cook for an additional 2-3 minutes, or until everything is well mixed and heated through.

6. **Serve:** Garnish with chopped green onions before serving.

Nutrients (per serving)

Calories: 320 kcal Carbohydrates: 45g Fiber: 6g

Protein: 14g Fat: 10g Sugar: 4g Sodium: 600mg

Calcium: 120mg

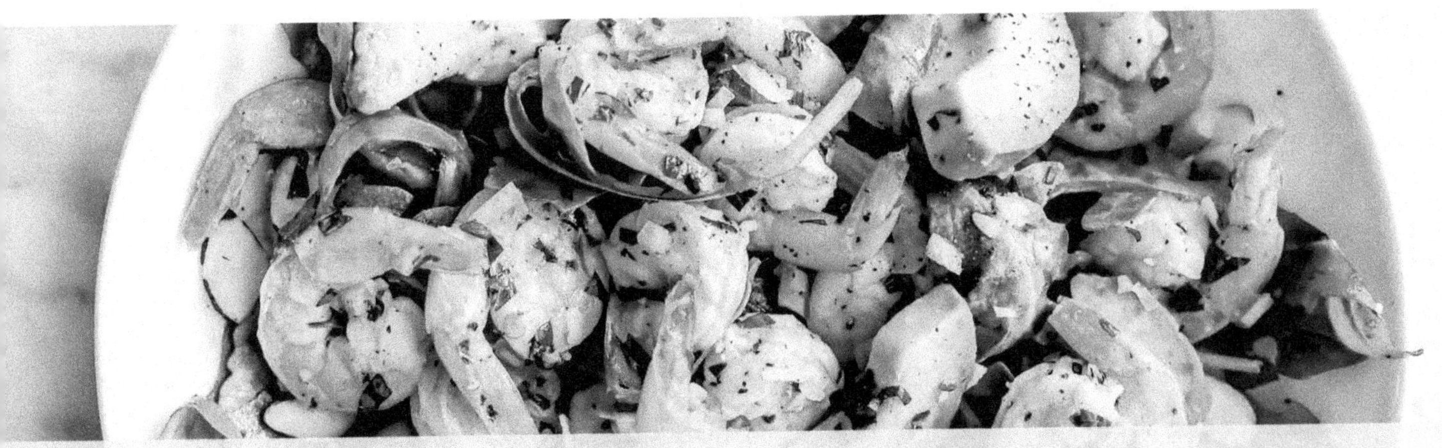

SHRIMP AND AVOCADO SALAD

Shrimp and Avocado Salad is a light, refreshing, and nutritious dish perfect for a quick lunch or dinner. The combination of succulent shrimp, creamy avocado, and crisp vegetables makes this salad both satisfying and healthful. It's low in calories yet high in flavor, thanks to the zesty dressing that ties all the ingredients together. This salad is also great for meal prepping, as it holds up well in the fridge.

Serves		**Preparation Time**		**Cooking Time**	
4		15 minutes		5 minute	

Ingredients:

1 lb (450g) large shrimp, peeled and deveined
1 tablespoon olive oil
1 teaspoon sucralose
1 teaspoon paprika
1/2 teaspoon garlic powder
Salt and pepper to taste
2 cups mixed salad greens
1 large avocado, diced
1 cup cherry tomatoes, halved
1/2 cucumber, sliced
1/4 red onion, thinly sliced
1/4 cup chopped fresh cilantro (for garnish)
For the Dressing:
2 tablespoons olive oil
1 tablespoon fresh lime juice
1 tablespoon apple cider vinegar
1 teaspoon sucralose
1/2 teaspoon cumin
Salt and pepper to taste

Instructions:

1. **Season and Cook Shrimp:** In a small bowl, mix together sucralose, paprika, garlic powder, salt, and pepper.Toss the shrimp in the spice mixture until evenly coated.Heat 1 tablespoon of olive oil in a large skillet over medium-high heat. Add the seasoned shrimp and cook for 2-3 minutes on each side, or until pink and opaque. Remove from heat and set aside.
2. **Prepare Salad:** In a large salad bowl, combine mixed salad greens, diced avocado, cherry tomatoes, cucumber, and red onion.
3. **Make Dressing:** In a small bowl, whisk together olive oil, lime juice, apple cider vinegar, sucralose, cumin, salt, and pepper.
4. **Assemble Salad:** Drizzle the dressing over the salad and toss to coat evenly.Top the salad with the cooked shrimp.
5. **Garnish and Serve:** Garnish with chopped fresh cilantro.Serve immediately.

Nutrients (per serving)

Calories: 270 kcal Carbohydrates: 14g Fiber: 7g

Protein: 23g Fat: 16g Sugar: 5g Sodium: 320mg

Calcium: 90mg

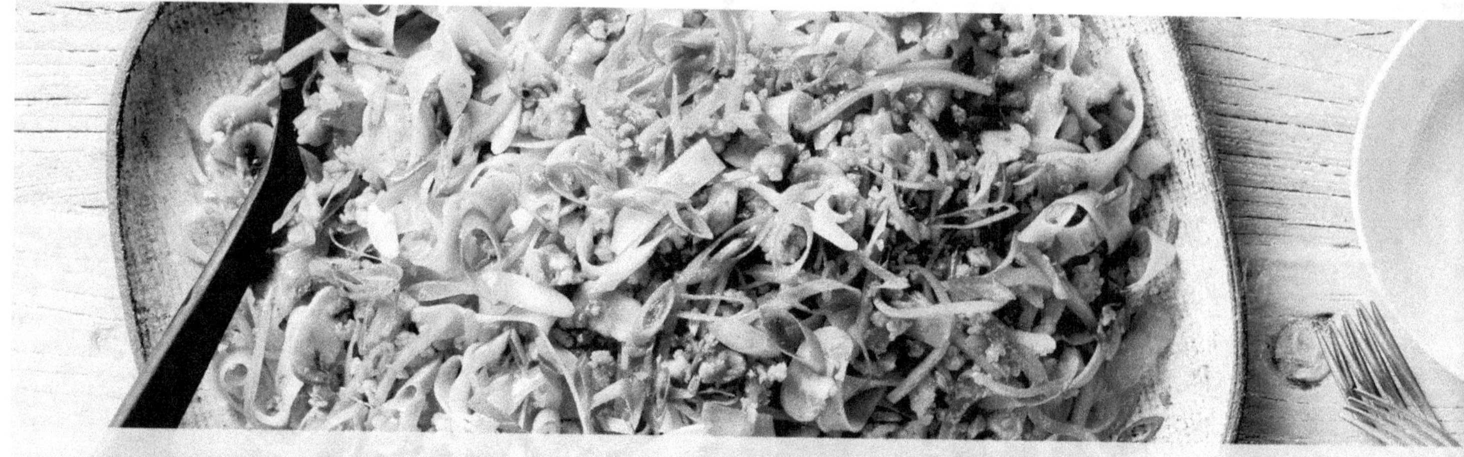

BROWN RICE NOODLES WITH CHICKEN AND VEGGIES

Brown Rice Noodles with Chicken and Veggies is a wholesome, flavorful dish that's perfect for a quick and nutritious meal. This recipe combines tender chicken, crisp vegetables, and chewy brown rice noodles in a savory sauce. It's an excellent choice for a balanced dinner, offering a good mix of protein, fiber, and essential nutrients. The dish is also adaptable, allowing you to use whatever vegetables you have on hand.

Serves	**Preparation Time**	**Cooking Time**
4 	15 minutes 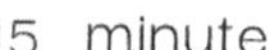	15 minute 

Ingredients:

- 8 oz (225g) brown rice noodles
- 1 tablespoon olive oil
- 1 lb (450g) chicken breast, thinly sliced
- 1 bell pepper, sliced
- 1 cup snap peas
- 1 cup broccoli florets
- 1 medium carrot, julienned
- 2 cloves garlic, minced
- 1 tablespoon fresh ginger, minced
- 1 tablespoon sucralose
- 3 tablespoons low-sodium soy sauce
- 2 tablespoons rice vinegar
- 1 tablespoon hoisin sauce
- 1 teaspoon sesame oil
- 1/4 cup chopped green onions (for garnish)
- 1 tablespoon sesame seeds (for garnish)

Instructions:

1. **Cook Noodles:** Cook the brown rice noodles according to package instructions. Drain and set aside.
2. **Cook Chicken:** Heat 2 tablespoons of olive oil in a large skillet or wok over medium-high heat. Add the sliced chicken and cook for 5-6 minutes, or until no longer pink and cooked through. Remove from the skillet and set aside.
3. **Stir-Fry Vegetables:** In the same skillet, add the bell pepper, snap peas, broccoli, and carrot. Stir-fry for 4-5 minutes, or until vegetables are tender-crisp. Add minced garlic and ginger to the vegetables and cook for an additional 1 minute.
4. **Combine Ingredients:** Return the cooked chicken to the skillet. Stir in sucralose, soy sauce, rice vinegar, hoisin sauce, and sesame oil. Toss to combine and heat through.
5. **Add Noodles:** Add the cooked brown rice noodles to the skillet and toss everything together until the noodles are evenly coated with the sauce.
6. **Garnish and Serve:** Garnish with chopped green onions and sesame seeds before serving.

Nutrients (per serving)

Calories: 320 kcal Carbohydrates: 45g Fiber: 5g

Protein: 25g Fat: 8g Sugar: 6g Sodium: 580mg

Calcium: 60mg

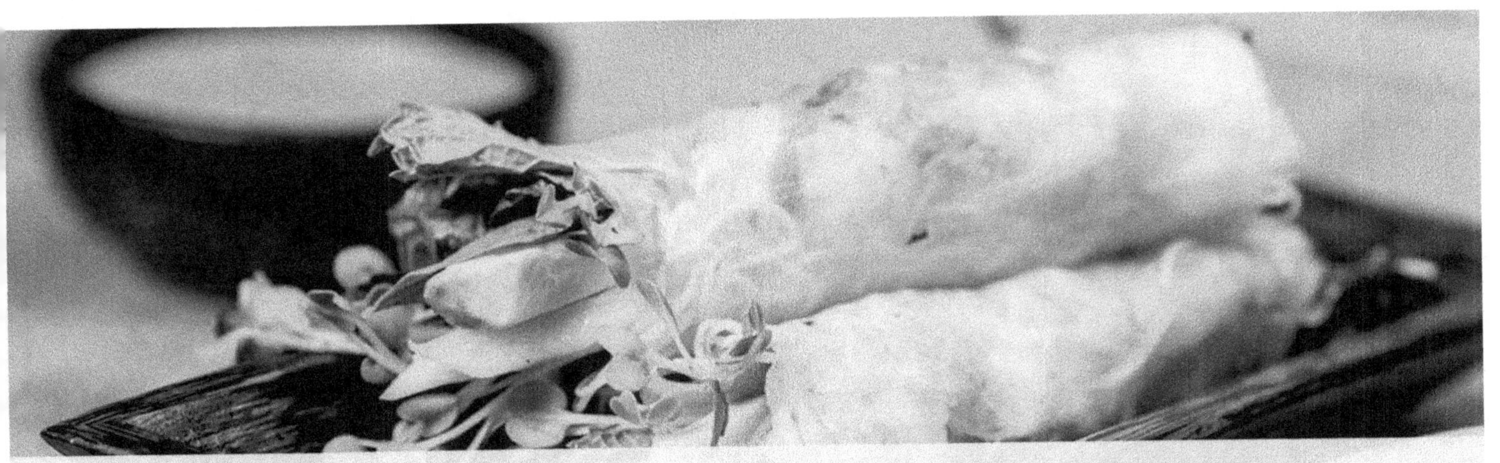

SHRIMP AND AVOCADO SPRING ROLLS

Shrimp and Avocado Spring Rolls are a fresh and vibrant choice for a light meal or appetizer. These rolls feature tender shrimp, creamy avocado, and crisp vegetables, all wrapped in delicate rice paper. They are perfect for a healthy, satisfying bite and can be served with a tangy dipping sauce for extra flavor. These spring rolls are low in calories and rich in nutrients, making them a great addition to your healthy meal prep routine.

Serves	Preparation Time	Cooking Time
4	20 minutes	5 minute

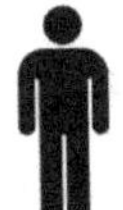  

Ingredients:

8 oz (225g) cooked shrimp, peeled and deveined

1 avocado, sliced

1 cup shredded carrots

1 cup cucumber, julienned

1 cup red bell pepper, thinly sliced

1 cup fresh basil leaves

1 cup fresh mint leaves

1 pack rice paper sheets (8-10 sheets)

1 tablespoon sucralose

3 tablespoons low-sodium soy sauce

2 tablespoons rice vinegar

1 tablespoon lime juice

1 teaspoon grated ginger

1 garlic clove, minced

Instructions:

1. **Prepare Rice Paper:** Fill a large bowl with warm water. Soak one rice paper sheet at a time in the water for about 10-15 seconds, or until it becomes pliable. Carefully remove and place on a clean surface.
2. **Assemble Spring Rolls:** On the lower third of the rice paper, arrange a few shrimp, avocado slices, shredded carrots, cucumber, red bell pepper, basil, and mint leaves.Sprinkle a small amount of sucralose over the filling.Fold the sides of the rice paper over the filling, then roll up from the bottom to form a tight roll. Repeat with the remaining ingredients.
3. **Prepare Dipping Sauce:** In a small bowl, whisk together soy sauce, rice vinegar, lime juice, grated ginger, and minced garlic.
4. **Serve:** Serve the spring rolls with the dipping sauce on the side.

Nutrients (per serving)

Calories: 150 kcal Carbohydrates: 22g Fiber: 4g

Protein: 10g Fat: 5g Sugar: 4g Sodium: 400mg

Calcium: 30mg

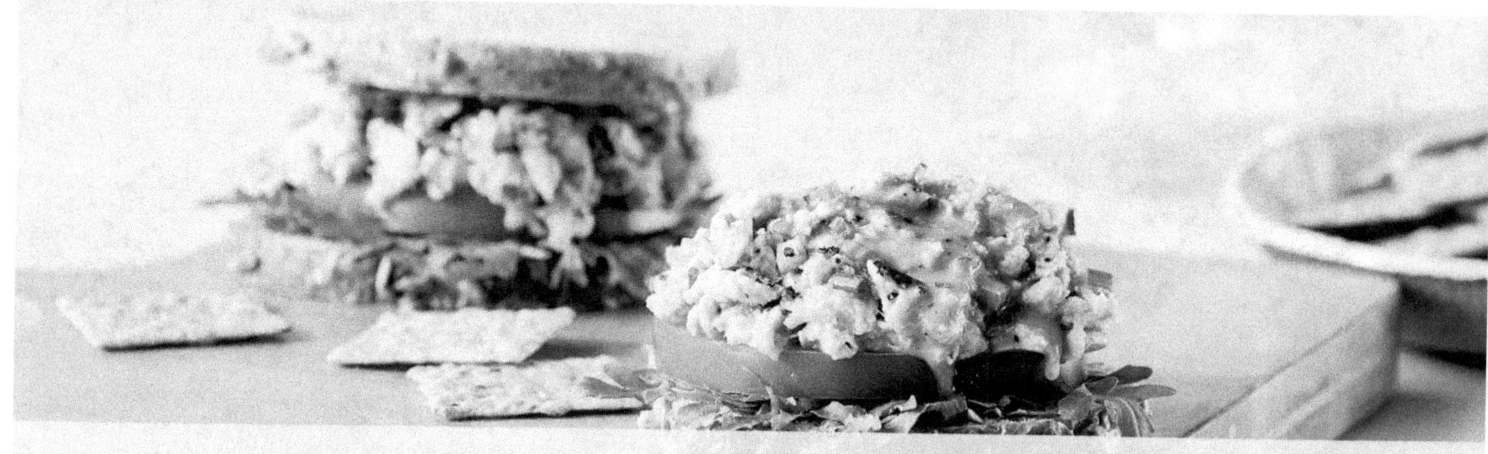

TUNA SALAD SANDWICH WITH FRESH GREENS

The Tuna Salad Sandwich with Fresh Greens is a wholesome and satisfying meal that's perfect for a quick lunch or a light dinner. This recipe combines protein-rich tuna with crisp greens and a creamy, flavorful dressing, all nestled between slices of whole-grain bread. It's not only delicious but also packed with nutrients, making it a great choice for a healthy meal prep.

Serves		**Preparation Time**		**Cooking Time**	
4		15 minutes		5 minute	

Ingredients:

2 cans (5 oz each) tuna in water, drained
1/4 cup Greek yogurt
1 tablespoon sucralose
2 tablespoons Dijon mustard
1 tablespoon lemon juice
1 celery stalk, finely chopped
1/4 cup red onion, finely chopped
2 tablespoons fresh parsley, chopped
8 slices whole-grain bread
2 cups mixed salad greens (e.g., lettuce, spinach, arugula)
Salt and pepper to taste

Instructions:

1. **Prepare Tuna Salad:** In a medium bowl, combine the drained tuna, Greek yogurt, sucralose, Dijon mustard, and lemon juice. Mix until well combined.Add the chopped celery, red onion, and parsley to the tuna mixture. Stir until evenly distributed. Season with salt and pepper to taste.
2. **Assemble Sandwiches:** Lay out 4 slices of whole-grain bread. Divide the tuna salad evenly among the bread slices.Top each sandwich with a generous handful of mixed salad greens.Place the remaining 4 slices of bread on top to complete the sandwiches.
3. **Serve:** Slice each sandwich in half and serve immediately, or wrap them up for a convenient lunch on the go.

Nutrients (per serving)

Calories: 320 kcal Carbohydrates: 30g Fiber: 5g
Protein: 25g Fat: 10g Sugar: 4g Sodium: 550mg
Calcium: 60mg

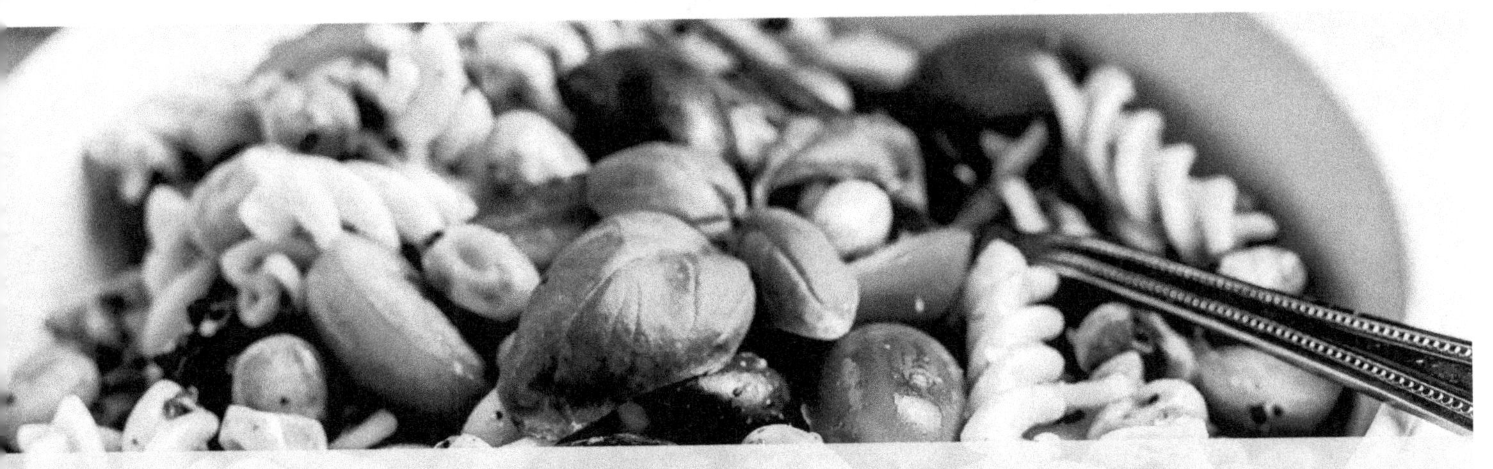

QUINOA PASTA WITH VEGGIES

Quinoa Pasta with Veggies is a vibrant and nutritious dish that combines the wholesome benefits of quinoa pasta with a medley of fresh vegetables. This meal is both gluten-free and packed with essential nutrients, making it an excellent choice for a healthy lunch or dinner. The light yet flavorful sauce and crunchy vegetables create a satisfying and wholesome meal that fits perfectly into any meal prep routine.

Serves		Preparation Time		Cooking Time	
4		10 minutes		20 minute	

Ingredients:

8 oz quinoa pasta

1 tablespoon olive oil

1 cup bell peppers, diced (red, yellow, or green)

1 cup zucchini, sliced

1 cup cherry tomatoes, halved

1 cup broccoli florets

3 cloves garlic, minced

1/4 cup fresh basil, chopped

1/4 cup grated Parmesan cheese (optional)

Salt and pepper to taste

1/2 teaspoon dried oregano

1/2 teaspoon dried thyme

Instructions:

1. **Cook Pasta:** Cook the quinoa pasta according to the package instructions. Drain and set aside.
2. **Sauté Vegetables:** In a large skillet, heat olive oil over medium heat.Add the garlic and sauté for about 1 minute until fragrant.Add the bell peppers, zucchini, cherry tomatoes, and broccoli to the skillet. Cook for 7-10 minutes, stirring occasionally, until the vegetables are tender.
3. **Season and Combine:** Season the vegetables with salt, pepper, dried oregano, and dried thyme. Stir to combine.Add the cooked quinoa pasta to the skillet and toss with the vegetables until well mixed and heated through.
4. **Finish and Serve:** Remove from heat and stir in the fresh basil.Serve hot, sprinkled with grated Parmesan cheese if desired.

Nutrients (per serving)

Calories: 320 kcal Carbohydrates: 45g Fiber: 6g

Protein: 12g Fat: 10g Sugar: 7g Sodium: 200mg

Calcium: 80mg

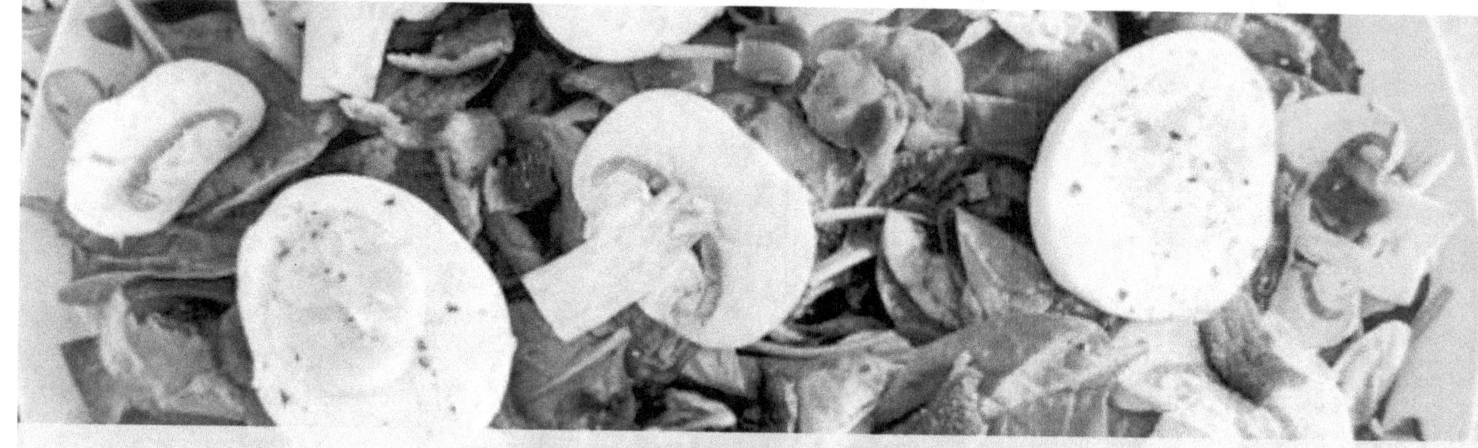

SPINACH SALAD WITH HARD-BOILED EGGS

Spinach Salad with Hard-Boiled Eggs is a refreshing and nutrient-packed dish that's perfect for a quick lunch or light dinner. This salad combines the rich, earthy flavor of fresh spinach with protein-rich hard-boiled eggs and a simple, tangy dressing. It's a balanced meal that provides essential vitamins and minerals while being both delicious and easy to prepare.

Serves 	**Preparation Time**	**Cooking Time** 
4	10 minutes	10 minute

Ingredients:

4 cups fresh spinach leaves
4 large eggs
1/2 cup cherry tomatoes, halved
1/4 cup red onion, thinly sliced
1/4 cup cucumber, sliced
1/4 cup crumbled feta cheese (optional)
2 tablespoons olive oil
1 tablespoon balsamic vinegar
1 teaspoon Dijon mustard
Salt and pepper to taste

Instructions:

1. **Prepare the Hard-Boiled Eggs:** Place eggs in a saucepan and cover with water. Bring to a boil over medium-high heat.Once boiling, cover the pan with a lid, remove from heat, and let the eggs sit for 9-10 minutes.Afterward, transfer the eggs to a bowl of ice water to cool. Once cooled, peel and slice them.
2. **Assemble the Salad:** In a large salad bowl, combine the fresh spinach leaves, cherry tomatoes, red onion, and cucumber. Top with sliced hard-boiled eggs and crumbled feta cheese if using.
3. **Prepare the Dressing:** In a small bowl, whisk together olive oil, balsamic vinegar, Dijon mustard, salt, and pepper. Drizzle the dressing over the salad and toss gently to coat.
4. **Serve:** Serve immediately or refrigerate for up to an hour before serving for a chilled option.

Nutrients (per serving)

Calories: 220 kcal Carbohydrates: 8g Fiber: 3g

Protein: 12g Fat: 16g Sugar: 4g Sodium: 250mg

Calcium: 150mg

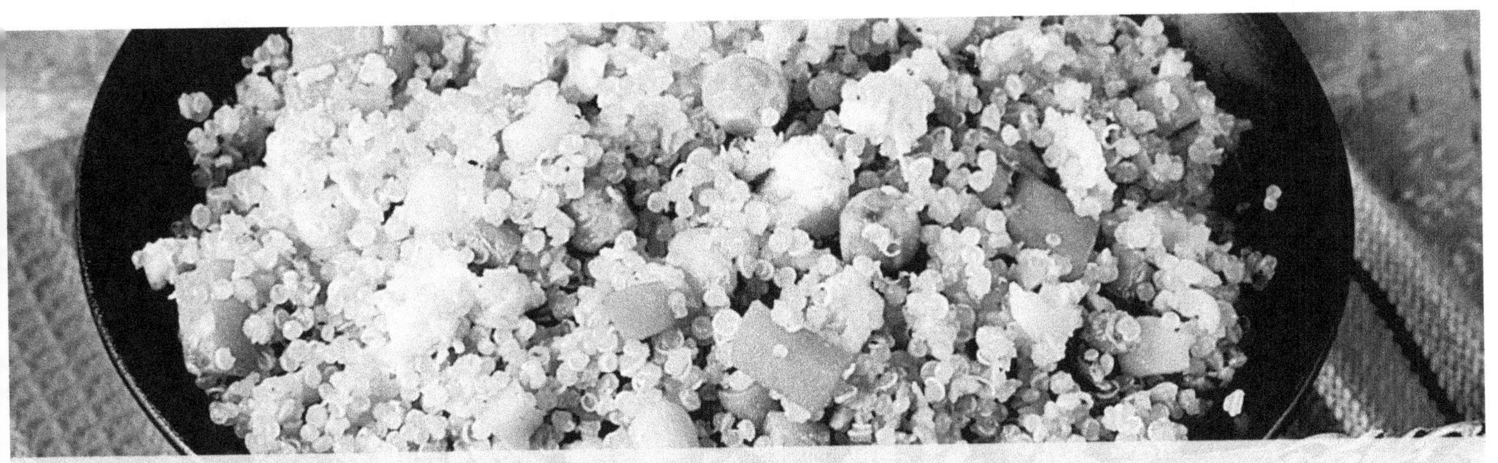

QUINOA FRIED RICE WITH VEGETABLES

Quinoa Fried Rice with Vegetables is a nutritious and flavorful twist on traditional fried rice. By substituting quinoa for rice, you boost the protein and fiber content while keeping the dish light and satisfying. Packed with colorful vegetables, this meal is both delicious and wholesome, making it perfect for lunch or dinner.

Serves 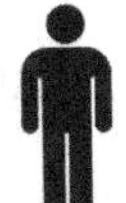	**Preparation Time** 	**Cooking Time** 
4	15 minutes	20 minute

Ingredients:

1 cup quinoa, uncooked
2 cups vegetable broth or water
2 tablespoons olive oil
1 small onion, diced
2 garlic cloves, minced
1/2 cup carrots, diced
1/2 cup bell peppers, diced
1/2 cup green peas (fresh or frozen)
1/2 cup broccoli florets
2 eggs, lightly beaten
2 tablespoons soy sauce (low-sodium)
1 tablespoon sesame oil
2 green onions, chopped
Salt and pepper to taste

Instructions:

1. **Cook the Quinoa:** Rinse quinoa under cold water. In a medium saucepan, bring 2 cups of vegetable broth or water to a boil. Add quinoa, reduce the heat, cover, and simmer for about 15 minutes or until all the liquid is absorbed and the quinoa is fluffy. Set aside.
2. **Prepare the Vegetables:** In a large skillet or wok, heat olive oil over medium heat. Add the diced onion and minced garlic, sautéing until fragrant (about 2-3 minutes). Add the diced carrots, bell peppers, green peas, and broccoli. Stir-fry for 5-7 minutes until the vegetables are tender yet crisp.
3. **Cook the Eggs:** Push the vegetables to one side of the skillet. Pour the beaten eggs into the other side and scramble them until fully cooked.
4. **Combine Everything:** Add the cooked quinoa to the skillet, stirring to combine with the vegetables and scrambled eggs. Pour in the soy sauce and sesame oil, mixing well. Cook for an additional 3-5 minutes, allowing the flavors to blend. Season with salt and pepper to taste.
5. **Garnish and Serve:** Remove from heat, sprinkle with chopped green onions, and serve hot.

Nutrients (per serving)

Calories: 280 kcal Carbohydrates: 30g Fiber: 6g

Protein: 10g Fat: 12g Sugar: 4g Sodium: 400mg

Calcium: 50mg

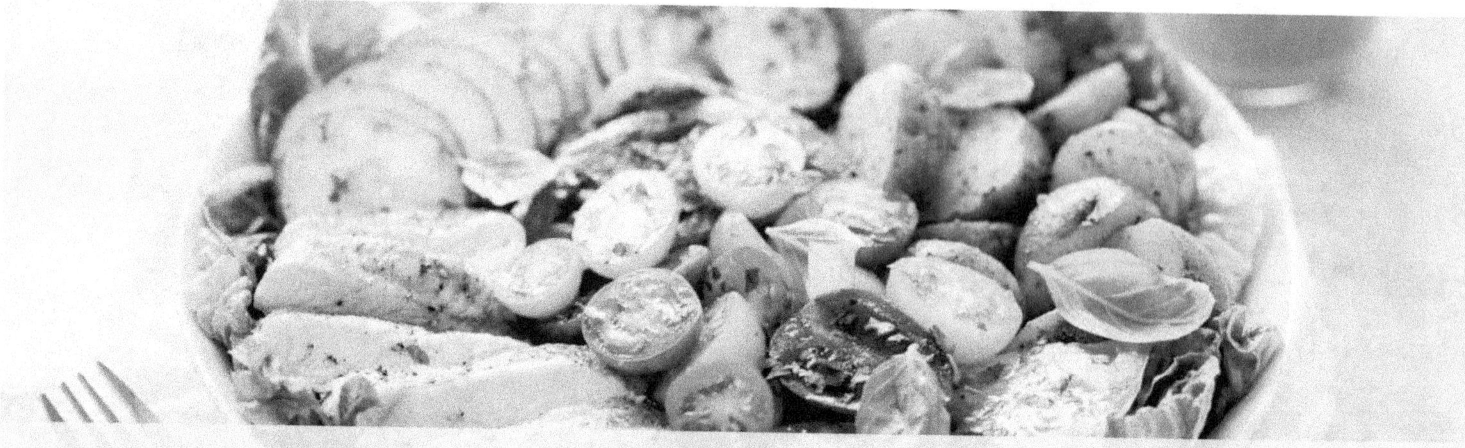

GRILLED CHICKEN WITH CUCUMBER SALAD

Grilled Chicken with Cucumber Salad is a light and refreshing meal perfect for a healthy lunch or dinner. The chicken is marinated with a simple mix of olive oil, herbs, and spices, while the cucumber salad offers a crisp and tangy balance. This dish is both nutritious and satisfying, making it a great option for meal prep or a quick, flavorful meal.

Serves		**Preparation Time**		**Cooking Time**	
4		15 minutes		20 minute	

Ingredients:

For the Chicken:

4 boneless, skinless chicken breasts

2 tablespoons olive oil

2 garlic cloves, minced

1 teaspoon dried oregano

1 teaspoon paprika

1 teaspoon salt

1/2 teaspoon black pepper

Juice of 1 lemon

For the Cucumber Salad:

2 large cucumbers, thinly sliced

1/2 red onion, thinly sliced

1/4 cup fresh dill, chopped

2 tablespoons olive oil

1 tablespoon white wine vinegar

Juice of 1 lemon

Salt and pepper to taste

Instructions:

1. **Marinate the Chicken:** In a small bowl, mix the olive oil, minced garlic, dried oregano, paprika, salt, pepper, and lemon juice. Place the chicken breasts in a resealable bag or shallow dish and pour the marinade over them. Let the chicken marinate for at least 15 minutes, or up to 2 hours in the refrigerator for more flavor.

2. **Grill the Chicken:** Preheat a grill or grill pan to medium-high heat.Grill the chicken for 6-7 minutes per side, or until fully cooked and the internal temperature reaches 165°F (74°C).Remove from the grill and let the chicken rest for a few minutes before serving.

3. **Prepare the Cucumber Salad:** In a large bowl, combine the sliced cucumbers, red onion, and chopped dill.In a small bowl, whisk together the olive oil, white wine vinegar, lemon juice, salt, and pepper.Pour the dressing over the cucumber mixture and toss to combine.

4. **Serve:** Plate the grilled chicken alongside the cucumber salad. Garnish with additional dill if desired.

Nutrients (per serving)

Calories: 280 kcal Carbohydrates: 6g Fiber: 2g

Protein: 32g Fat: 14g Sugar: 3g Sodium: 450mg

Calcium: 30mg

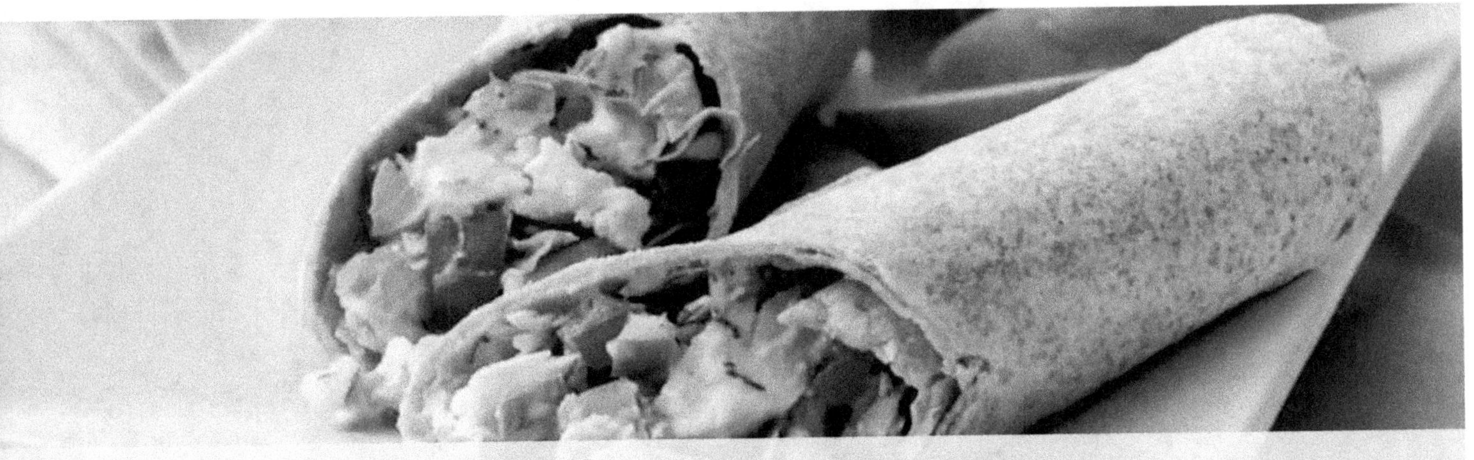

TUNA WRAP WITH CUCUMBER

Tuna Wrap with Cucumber is a light, refreshing, and protein-packed meal perfect for lunch or a quick snack. The combination of creamy tuna salad, crisp cucumbers, and whole grain wraps offers a nutritious, balanced meal that's easy to make and perfect for meal prep. It's a great option for those looking for a satisfying yet healthy dish that can be enjoyed on the go.

Serves		**Preparation Time**		**Cooking Time**	
4		10 minutes	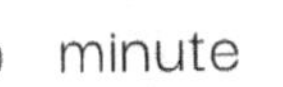	0 minute	

Ingredients:

2 cans (5 oz each) of tuna in water, drained

1/4 cup plain Greek yogurt

1 tablespoon mayonnaise

1 tablespoon Dijon mustard

1/2 cucumber, thinly sliced

1/4 red onion, finely chopped

1 tablespoon fresh dill, chopped (optional)

Salt and pepper to taste

4 whole grain wraps

1 cup mixed greens

Instructions:

1. **Prepare the Tuna Salad:** In a medium bowl, mix the drained tuna, Greek yogurt, mayonnaise, Dijon mustard, red onion, and fresh dill. Season with salt and pepper to taste. Stir until well combined.
2. **Assemble the Wraps:** Lay out the whole grain wraps on a clean surface.Spread a quarter of the tuna salad evenly onto each wrap.Add cucumber slices and a handful of mixed greens on top of the tuna.
3. **Wrap and Serve:** Roll up each wrap tightly, folding in the sides as you go.Slice in half, if desired, and serve immediately, or wrap in foil or plastic wrap to enjoy later.

Nutrients (per serving)

Calories: 260 kcal Carbohydrates: 22g Fiber: 4g

Protein: 23g Fat: 10g Sugar: 2g Sodium: 450mg

Calcium: 50mg

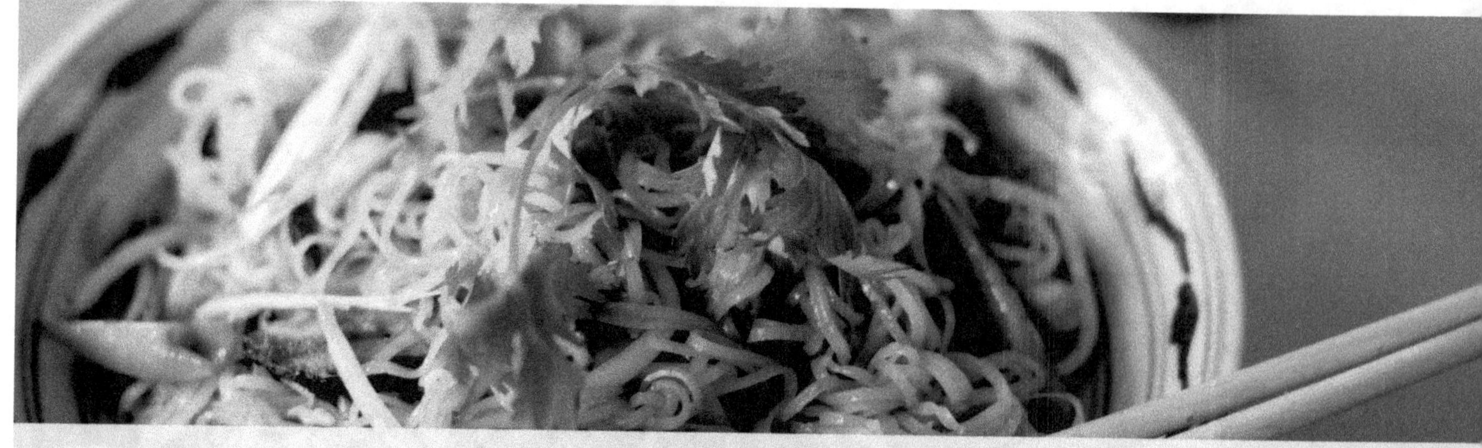

BROWN RICE NOODLES WITH CHICKEN AND SPINACH

Brown Rice Noodles with Chicken and Spinach is a wholesome and flavorful dish that combines tender chicken, nutrient-rich spinach, and hearty brown rice noodles. This recipe is perfect for a quick and satisfying weeknight dinner while offering a good balance of protein, fiber, and vitamins. It's a gluten-free option that doesn't compromise on taste or nutrition.

Serves		**Preparation Time**		**Cooking Time**	
4		10 minutes		20 minute	

Ingredients:

8 oz brown rice noodles

2 tablespoons olive oil

2 chicken breasts, sliced thinly

2 garlic cloves, minced

1 tablespoon soy sauce (low sodium)

1 tablespoon sucralose

1/4 teaspoon red pepper flakes (optional)

4 cups fresh spinach leaves

1 tablespoon lemon juice

Salt and pepper to taste

2 tablespoons sesame seeds for garnish (optional)

Instructions:

1. **Cook the Noodles:** Boil water in a large pot and cook the brown rice noodles according to the package instructions. Drain and set aside.
2. **Cook the Chicken:** Heat 1 tablespoon of olive oil in a large skillet over medium heat. Add the sliced chicken breasts and season with salt and pepper. Cook for 5-7 minutes, or until the chicken is browned and cooked through. Remove the chicken from the pan and set aside.
3. **Sauté Garlic and Spinach:** In the same skillet, add the remaining tablespoon of olive oil. Add the minced garlic and sauté for 1 minute until fragrant.Add the spinach leaves and cook for 2-3 minutes, stirring frequently, until wilted.
4. **Combine Everything:** Return the chicken to the skillet with the spinach. Add the cooked brown rice noodles, soy sauce, sucralose, red pepper flakes (if using), and lemon juice.Toss everything together and cook for an additional 2-3 minutes until the ingredients are well combined and heated through.
5. **Serve:** Divide the noodle mixture among four bowls. Garnish with sesame seeds, if desired, and serve immediately.

Nutrients (per serving)

Calories: 370 kcal Carbohydrates: 45g Fiber: 5g

Protein: 28g Fat: 10g Sugar: 1g Sodium: 350mg

Calcium: 70mg

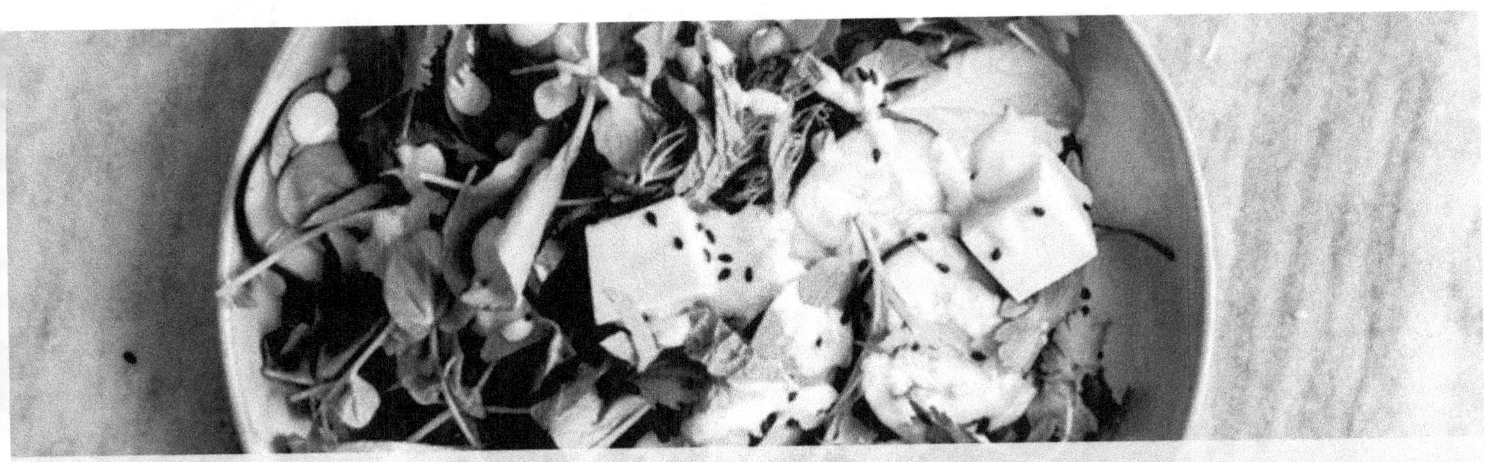

TOFU AND GREEN VEGETABLE SALAD

This Tofu and Green Vegetable Salad is a refreshing and nutritious dish that combines crispy tofu with a variety of green vegetables. It's a plant-based meal rich in protein, fiber, and essential vitamins. This salad is perfect for a light lunch or dinner, offering a flavorful way to enjoy wholesome ingredients.

Serves		**Preparation Time**		**Cooking Time**	
4		10 minutes		15 minute	

Ingredients:

1 block (14 oz) firm tofu, pressed and cubed

1 tablespoon olive oil

1 cucumber, diced

1 cup green beans, blanched

2 cups fresh spinach leaves

1/2 cup broccoli florets, steamed

1 avocado, sliced

2 tablespoons sucralose

2 tablespoons soy sauce (low sodium)

1 tablespoon rice vinegar

1 tablespoon sesame oil

1 tablespoon sesame seeds for garnish

Salt and pepper to taste

Instructions:

1. **Prepare the Tofu:** Heat olive oil in a skillet over medium heat. Add the cubed tofu and cook for 7-10 minutes, flipping occasionally until golden brown on all sides. Season with salt and pepper. Remove from heat and set aside.

2. **Blanch and Steam Vegetables:** Blanch the green beans by boiling them for 2-3 minutes, then immediately transferring them to ice-cold water to preserve their color and crispness. Steam the broccoli florets for 3-5 minutes until tender but still vibrant green.

3. **Assemble the Salad:** In a large bowl, combine the spinach leaves, cucumber, blanched green beans, and steamed broccoli. Add the tofu and avocado slices.

4. **Prepare the Dressing:** In a small bowl, whisk together the sucralose, soy sauce, rice vinegar, and sesame oil.

5. **Dress the Salad:** Drizzle the dressing over the salad and toss gently to coat all the ingredients evenly.

6. **Serve:** Divide the salad among four plates and sprinkle with sesame seeds before serving.

Nutrients (per serving)

Calories: 280 kcal Carbohydrates: 15g Fiber: 6g

Protein: 15g Fat: 18g Sugar: 2g Sodium: 430mg

Calcium: 150mg

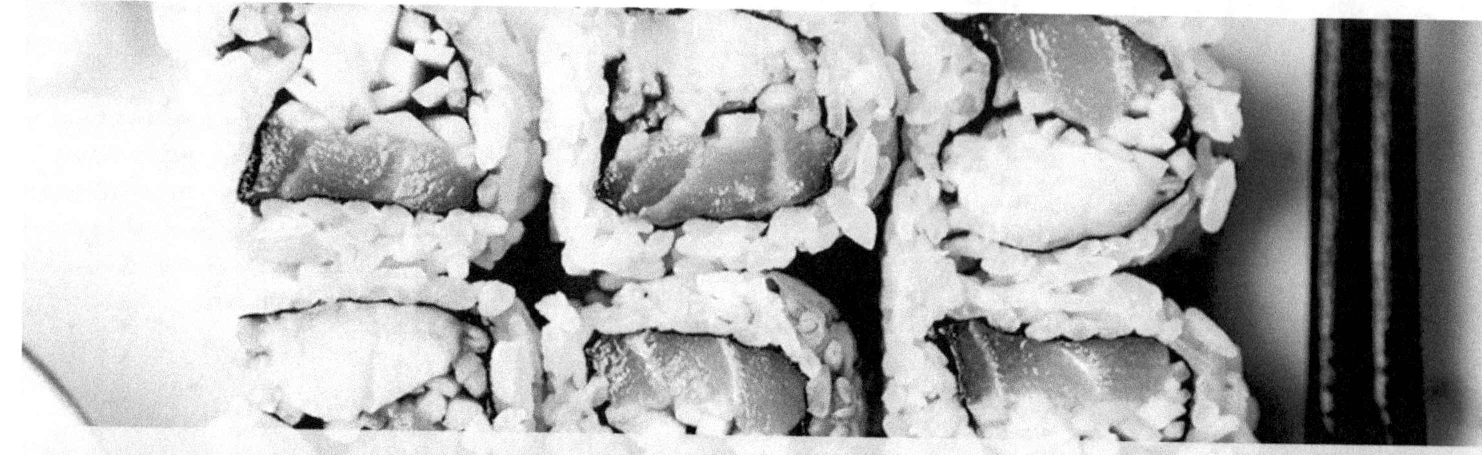

SALMON AND AVOCADO SUSHI ROLLS

Salmon and Avocado Sushi Rolls are a simple and delicious way to enjoy sushi at home. These rolls combine the creamy richness of avocado with the fresh, buttery taste of salmon. This healthy meal is packed with heart-healthy omega-3 fatty acids from the salmon and a dose of fiber from the avocado. Perfect for lunch or dinner, these sushi rolls are a nutritious, satisfying option that can be enjoyed by sushi lovers and beginners alike.

Serves 	**Preparation Time** 	**Cooking Time** 
4	20 minutes	15 minute

Ingredients:

2 cups sushi rice
2 1/2 cups water
2 tablespoons rice vinegar
1 tablespoon sucralose
1/2 teaspoon salt
8 oz fresh salmon, thinly sliced
1 avocado, sliced
4 sheets nori (seaweed)
Soy sauce (for serving)
Pickled ginger (for serving)
Wasabi (optional)

Instructions:

1. **Cook the Rice:** Rinse the sushi rice under cold water until the water runs clear. In a medium saucepan, combine the rice and water, and bring to a boil. Lower the heat, cover, and simmer for 15 minutes, or until the rice is fully cooked. Remove from heat and let it sit for 10 minutes, covered.
2. **Season the Rice:** In a small bowl, mix the rice vinegar, sucralose, and salt. Gently fold this mixture into the cooked rice until well combined. Allow the rice to cool slightly.
3. **Prepare the Ingredients:** Thinly slice the salmon and avocado. Set aside.
4. **Assemble the Sushi Rolls:** Lay a sheet of nori on a bamboo sushi mat, shiny side down. Wet your hands with water to prevent the rice from sticking. Spread an even layer of sushi rice over the nori, leaving about 1 inch of space at the top edge. Arrange a few slices of salmon and avocado along the center of the rice. Roll the sushi tightly, starting from the bottom edge, using the bamboo mat to guide you. Press firmly to seal the roll.
5. **Slice and Serve:** Using a sharp knife, slice the sushi roll into bite-sized pieces. Repeat the process with the remaining nori sheets, rice, salmon, and avocado.
6. **Serve:** Serve the sushi rolls with soy sauce, pickled ginger, and wasabi, if desired.

Nutrients (per serving)

Calories: 320 kcal Carbohydrates: 40g Fiber: 4g
Protein: 18g Fat: 12g Sugar: 1g Sodium: 270mg
Calcium: 25mg

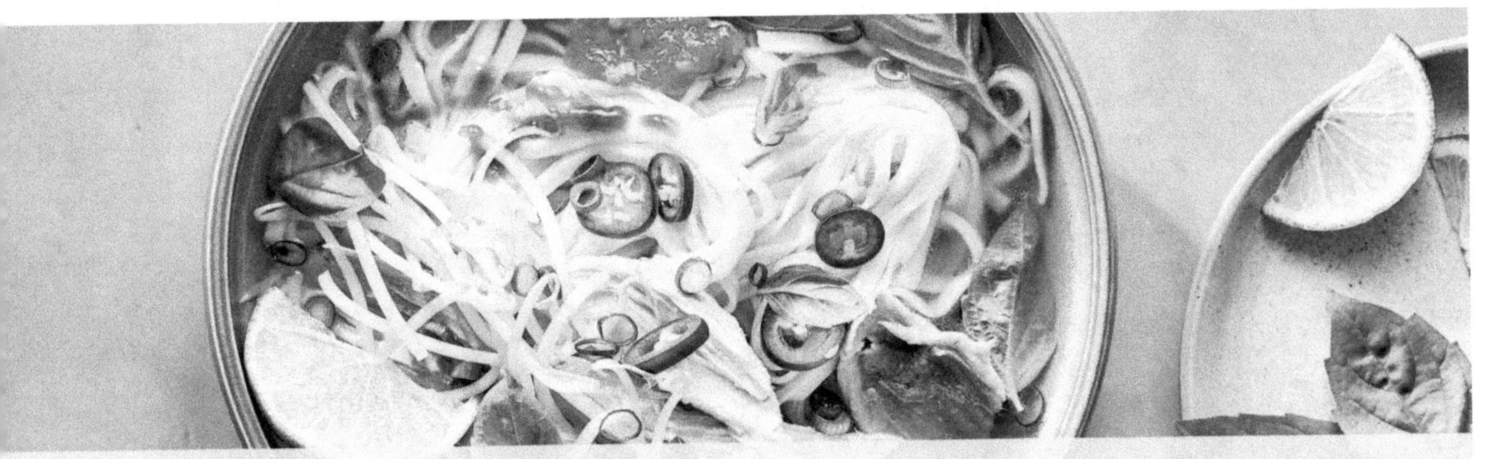

FRESH CHICKEN PHO

Fresh Chicken Pho is a light yet flavorful Vietnamese soup that combines tender chicken with fragrant herbs and rice noodles in a deliciously savory broth. This wholesome dish is perfect for a healthy lunch or dinner, offering a balance of lean protein, fresh vegetables, and aromatic spices. It's low in fat and packed with nutrients, making it a great choice for anyone looking to enjoy a nutritious, comforting meal.

Serves	**Preparation Time**	**Cooking Time**
4	20 minutes	1 hour

Ingredients:

For the Broth:

1 lb chicken breast (bone-in for more flavor)

1 large onion, halved

1 piece (2-inch) fresh ginger, sliced

1 cinnamon stick

2 star anise

4 cloves

8 cups chicken broth (low sodium)

2 tablespoons fish sauce

1 tablespoon sucralose (optional, for sweetness)

Salt, to taste

For the Soup:

8 oz rice noodles

2 cups bean sprouts

1 cup fresh cilantro leaves

1 cup fresh basil leaves

1/2 cup sliced green onions

1 lime, cut into wedges

1 fresh jalapeño, sliced (optional)

Instructions:

1. **Prepare the Broth:** In a large pot, toast the onion and ginger over medium heat until lightly charred, about 5 minutes. Add the cinnamon stick, star anise, and cloves, and toast for 2 minutes to release the aromas. Pour in the chicken broth, add the chicken breast, fish sauce, sucralose, and salt. Bring to a boil, then reduce the heat to low and simmer for 45 minutes. Once the chicken is fully cooked, remove it from the broth and shred the meat. Set aside. Strain the broth to remove the spices and vegetables, then return the broth to the pot.
2. **Cook the Noodles:** While the broth is simmering, cook the rice noodles according to the package instructions. Drain and set aside.
3. **Assemble the Pho:** Divide the cooked noodles among 4 bowls. Top each bowl with shredded chicken, bean sprouts, cilantro, basil, and green onions. Ladle the hot broth over the noodles and toppings. Serve with lime wedges and jalapeño slices for extra flavor.

Nutrients (per serving)

Calories: 310 kcal Carbohydrates: 40g Fiber: 3g

Protein: 28g Fat: 6g Sugar: 4g Sodium: 900mg

Calcium: 70mg

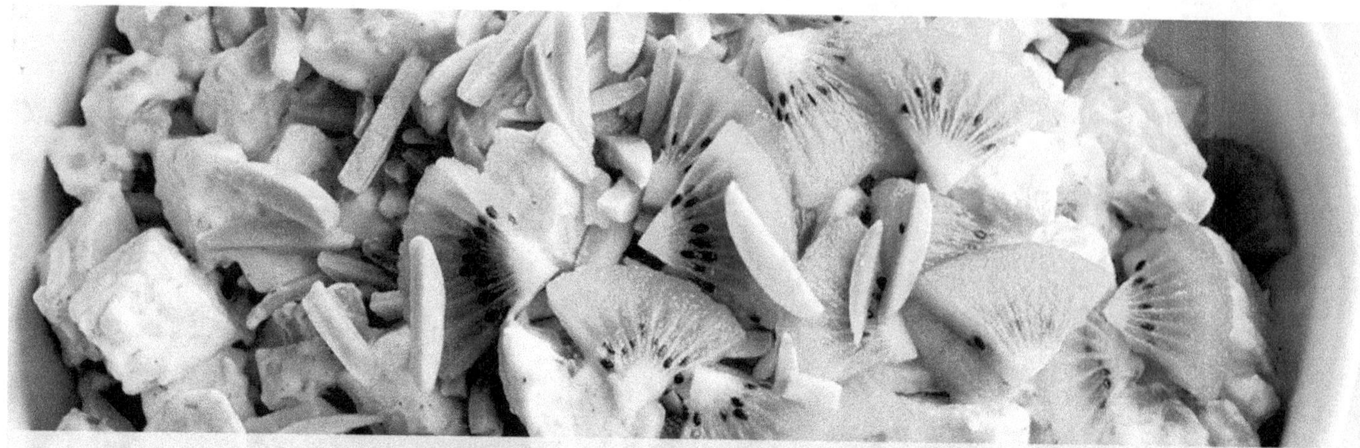

ALMOND CHICKEN SALAD

Almond Chicken Salad is a light, protein-packed dish perfect for a healthy lunch or dinner. This salad combines tender grilled chicken with crunchy almonds and fresh greens, offering a delightful mix of textures and flavors. It's rich in lean protein, healthy fats, and essential vitamins, making it both nutritious and satisfying.

Serves	 Preparation Time	 Cooking Time	
4	20 minutes	15 minutes	

Ingredients:

2 chicken breasts, boneless and skinless
1/4 cup slivered almonds, toasted
6 cups mixed greens (spinach, arugula, and lettuce)
1 cup cherry tomatoes, halved
1/2 cup cucumber, sliced
1/4 cup red onion, thinly sliced
1 avocado, diced
1/4 cup feta cheese (optional)
2 tablespoons olive oil
1 tablespoon lemon juice
1 tablespoon sucralose (optional, for sweetness)
Salt and pepper, to taste

Instructions:

1. **Cook the Chicken:** Season the chicken breasts with salt and pepper. Heat 1 tablespoon of olive oil in a skillet over medium heat. Cook the chicken for 6-7 minutes per side, or until fully cooked. Remove from the skillet, let it cool slightly, then slice into strips.
2. **Prepare the Salad:** In a large salad bowl, combine the mixed greens, cherry tomatoes, cucumber, red onion, and avocado. Add the sliced chicken and toasted almonds on top. If using, sprinkle the salad with feta cheese.
3. **Make the Dressing:** In a small bowl, whisk together the remaining olive oil, lemon juice, sucralose, salt, and pepper. Drizzle the dressing over the salad and toss gently to combine.
4. **Serve:** Divide the salad into 4 servings and enjoy fresh.

Nutrients (per serving)

Calories: 320 kcal Carbohydrates: 10g Fiber: 6g
Protein: 28g Fat: 19g Sugar: 3g Sodium: 220mg
Calcium: 80mg

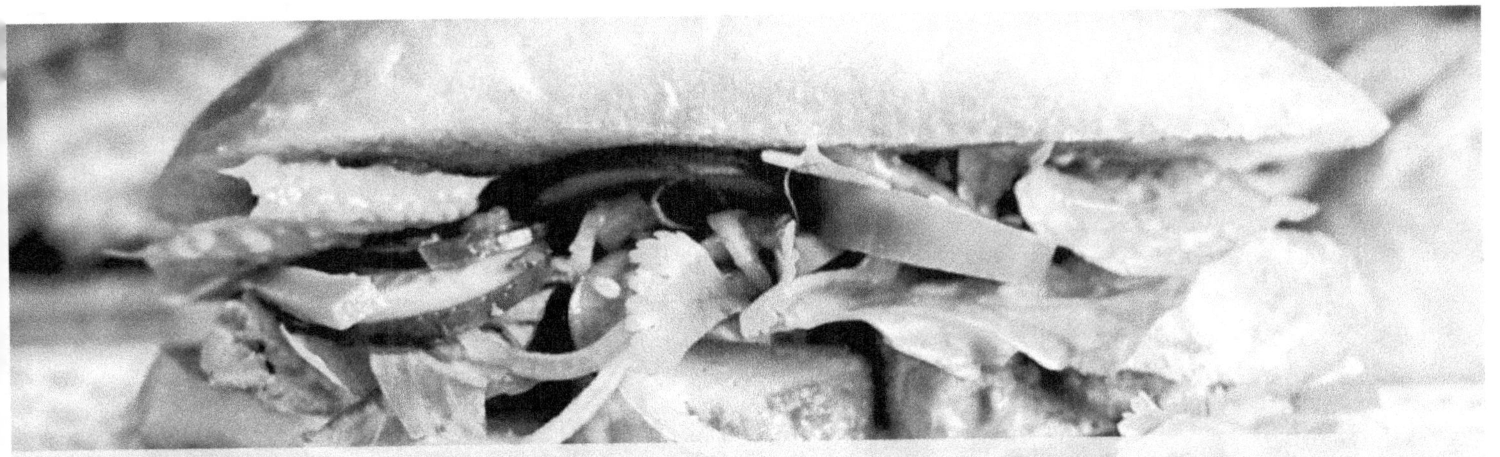

PORK BANH MI SANDWICH WITH FRESH VEGETABLES

The Pork Banh Mi Sandwich is a classic Vietnamese street food dish that blends savory, marinated pork with fresh, crisp vegetables in a light, airy baguette. This recipe adds a healthy twist by using sucralose to sweeten the marinade. It's packed with flavor, combining the tanginess of pickled veggies, the richness of pork, and the freshness of herbs for a well-balanced meal.

Serves		Preparation Time		Cooking Time	
4		20 minutes		15 minutes	

Ingredients:

1 lb pork tenderloin, thinly sliced

1 baguette (or 4 small baguettes)

1/4 cup soy sauce

1 tablespoon sucralose

1 tablespoon fish sauce

1 tablespoon rice vinegar

2 cloves garlic, minced

1/2 teaspoon black pepper

1/4 cup mayonnaise (optional)

1 tablespoon sriracha or hot sauce (optional)

For the Pickled Vegetables:

1/2 cup carrots, julienned

1/2 cup daikon radish, julienned

1/2 cup cucumber, thinly sliced

1/4 cup rice vinegar

1 tablespoon sucralose

1/2 teaspoon salt

1/4 cup water

For Garnish:

Fresh cilantro

Sliced jalapeños (optional)

Instructions:

1. **Prepare the Pickled Vegetables:** In a bowl, mix rice vinegar, sucralose, salt, and water. Add the julienned carrots, daikon radish, and cucumber. Let it sit for 15-20 minutes to pickle.
2. **Marinate the Pork:** In a separate bowl, combine soy sauce, fish sauce, rice vinegar, minced garlic, black pepper, and sucralose. Add the pork slices to the marinade and let it sit for 15 minutes.
3. **Cook the Pork:** Heat a skillet or grill pan over medium heat. Cook the marinated pork slices for about 3-4 minutes per side, until fully cooked and caramelized.
4. **Prepare the Baguettes:** Slice the baguettes open lengthwise, leaving one side connected. If using, spread mayonnaise and sriracha inside the baguettes.
5. **Assemble the Sandwiches:** Add a layer of cooked pork to the bottom of each baguette. Drain the pickled vegetables and layer them on top of the pork. Add fresh cilantro and jalapeño slices for garnish.
6. **Serve:** Cut each sandwich in half and serve immediately.

Nutrients (per serving)

Calories: 390 kcal Carbohydrates: 36g Fiber: 3g

Protein: 28g Fat: 13g Sugar: 4g Sodium: 700mg

Calcium: 50mg

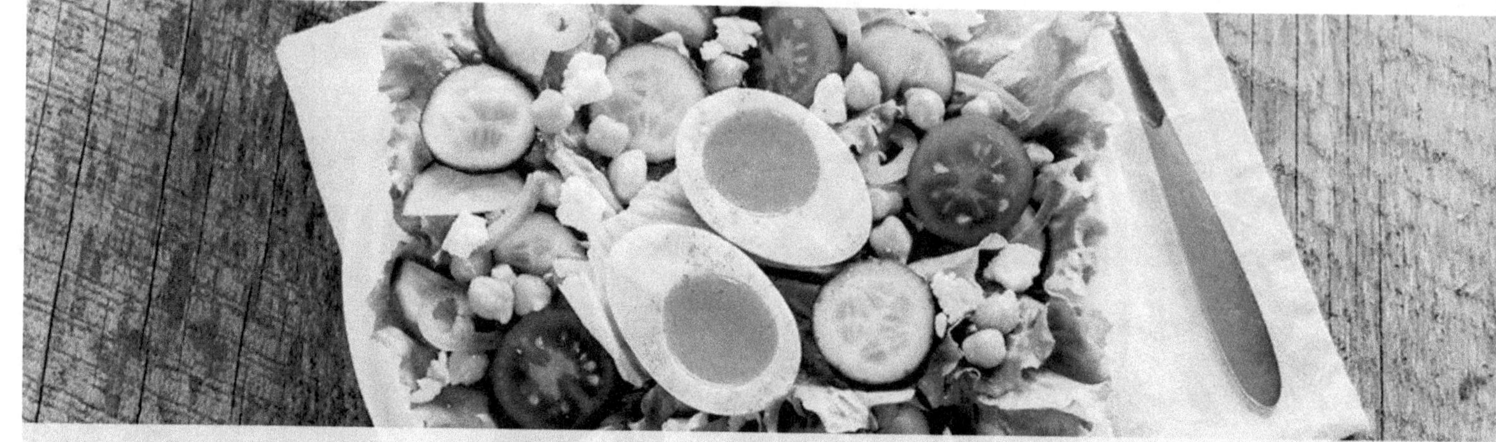

MIXED VEGGIE SALAD WITH HARD-BOILED EGGS

This Mixed Veggie Salad with Hard-Boiled Eggs is a nutrient-packed, vibrant meal that combines fresh, crisp vegetables with protein-rich eggs. Ideal for a light lunch or a wholesome dinner, this salad features a delightful blend of textures and flavors, enhanced with a simple, tangy dressing. It's a great way to enjoy a variety of vegetables while keeping your meal satisfying and nutritious.

Serves
4

Preparation Time
15 minutes

Cooking Time
10 minutes

Ingredients:

4 large eggs
1 cup cherry tomatoes, halved
1 cup cucumber, diced
1 cup bell peppers (red, yellow, or orange), diced
1 cup shredded carrots
1 cup baby spinach leaves
1/4 cup red onion, thinly sliced
1/4 cup fresh parsley, chopped
For the Dressing:
3 tablespoons olive oil
2 tablespoons balsamic vinegar
1 tablespoon lemon juice
1 teaspoon sucralose
1 teaspoon Dijon mustard
Salt and pepper to taste

Instructions:

1. **Cook the Quinoa:** In a medium saucepan, bring the vegetable broth or water to a boil. Add the quinoa, reduce the heat to low, cover, and simmer for 15 minutes, or until the liquid is absorbed and the quinoa is tender. Fluff with a fork and set aside.
2. **Prepare the Stir-Fry:** Heat olive oil in a large skillet or wok over medium-high heat. Add garlic and ginger and sauté for 1 minute until fragrant. Add bell peppers, broccoli, snap peas, carrots, and mushrooms. Stir-fry for 5-7 minutes until the vegetables are tender-crisp.
3. **Combine and Season:** Add the cooked quinoa to the skillet with the vegetables and stir to combine. Stir in soy sauce and sucralose, and cook for an additional 2-3 minutes, allowing the flavors to meld.
4. **Serve:** Remove from heat and garnish with sliced green onions and sesame seeds, if desired. Divide the stir-fry among four plates and serve immediately.

Nutrients (per serving)

Calories: 320 kcal Carbohydrates: 45g Fiber: 6g
Protein: 11g Fat: 8g Sugar: 7g Sodium: 600mg
Calcium: 80mg

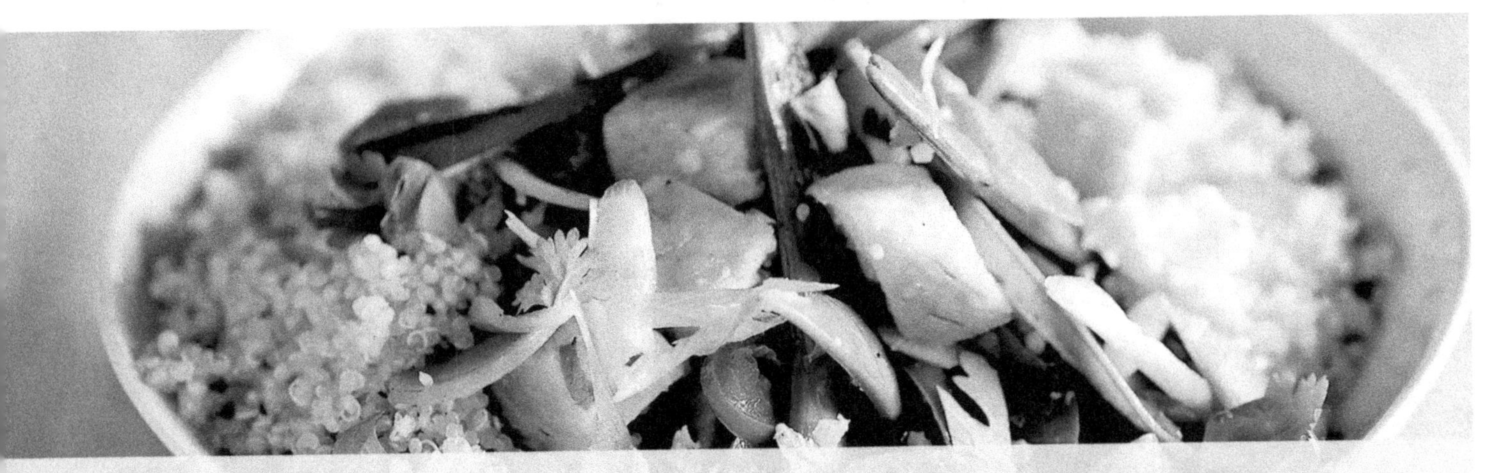

QUINOA STIR-FRY WITH VEGETABLES

Quinoa Stir-Fry with Vegetables is a versatile, colorful dish that combines protein-packed quinoa with a variety of fresh, crisp vegetables. This quick and easy recipe is perfect for a nutritious lunch or dinner, offering a delightful mix of textures and flavors. It's a fantastic option for meal prep, ensuring you have a healthy, satisfying meal ready in no time.

Serves	Preparation Time	Cooking Time
4	15 minutes	20 minutes

Ingredients:

1 cup quinoa, rinsed

2 cups vegetable broth or water

1 tablespoon olive oil

1 cup bell peppers (red, yellow, or green), diced

1 cup broccoli florets

1 cup snap peas

1 cup carrots, thinly sliced

1 cup mushrooms, sliced

2 cloves garlic, minced

1 tablespoon fresh ginger, minced

2 tablespoons low-sodium soy sauce

1 tablespoon sucralose

2 green onions, sliced

1 tablespoon sesame seeds (optional)

Instructions:

1. **Prepare the Hard-Boiled Eggs:** Place the eggs in a saucepan and cover them with water. Bring to a boil over medium-high heat, then reduce the heat and simmer for 10 minutes. Remove the eggs and place them in a bowl of ice water to cool. Once cooled, peel and slice them.
2. **Prepare the Salad:** In a large salad bowl, combine cherry tomatoes, cucumber, bell peppers, shredded carrots, baby spinach, red onion, and fresh parsley.
3. **Prepare the Dressing:** In a small bowl or jar, whisk together olive oil, balsamic vinegar, lemon juice, sucralose, Dijon mustard, salt, and pepper until well combined.
4. **Assemble the Salad:** Pour the dressing over the salad and toss to coat the vegetables evenly. Top the salad with sliced hard-boiled eggs.
5. **Serve:** Divide the salad among four plates and serve immediately.

Nutrients (per serving)

Calories: 250 kcal Carbohydrates: 12g Fiber: 4g

Protein: 14g Fat: 16g Sugar: 5g Sodium: 320mg

Calcium: 90mg

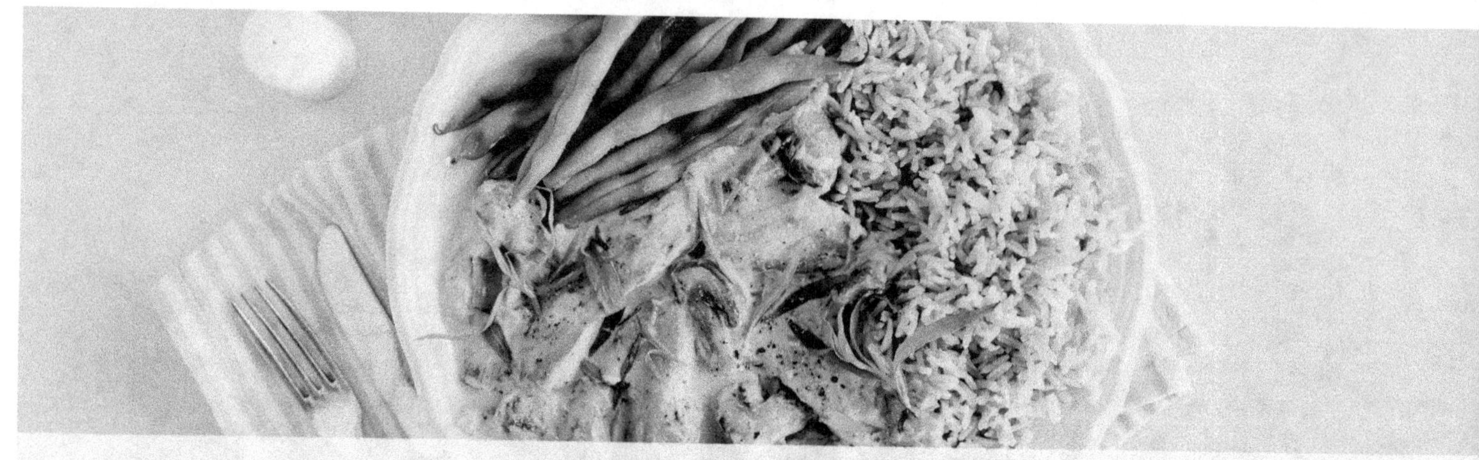

BROWN RICE PASTA WITH CHICKEN AND GREENS

Brown Rice Pasta with Chicken and Greens is a wholesome and satisfying meal that combines the nutty flavor of brown rice pasta with tender chicken and a mix of fresh greens. This dish is not only delicious but also packed with nutrients, making it an excellent choice for a healthy lunch or dinner. The light sauce and vibrant vegetables enhance the overall flavor while keeping the meal balanced and nutritious.

Serves	 **Preparation Time**	 **Cooking Time**	
4	15 minutes	25 minutes	

Ingredients:

8 ounces brown rice pasta

2 tablespoons olive oil

1 pound chicken breast, cut into bite-sized pieces

2 cloves garlic, minced

1 cup spinach leaves

1 cup kale, chopped

1 cup zucchini, sliced

1 cup cherry tomatoes, halved

1 tablespoon low-sodium soy sauce

1 tablespoon sucralose

1 teaspoon dried oregano

Salt and pepper to taste

2 tablespoons grated Parmesan cheese (optional)

Instructions:

1. **Cook the Pasta:** Bring a large pot of salted water to a boil. Add the brown rice pasta and cook according to package instructions, usually 7-9 minutes, until al dente. Drain and set aside.

2. **Prepare the Chicken:** Heat olive oil in a large skillet over medium-high heat.Add chicken pieces and cook for 5-7 minutes, or until fully cooked and golden brown. Remove the chicken from the skillet and set aside.

3. **Cook the Vegetables:** In the same skillet, add minced garlic and sauté for 1 minute until fragrant.Add spinach, kale, zucchini, and cherry tomatoes. Cook for 5-7 minutes, stirring occasionally, until the vegetables are tender and the greens are wilted.

4. **Combine and Season:** Return the cooked chicken to the skillet and stir to combine with the vegetables.Add the cooked brown rice pasta to the skillet.Stir in soy sauce, sucralose, dried oregano, salt, and pepper. Cook for an additional 2-3 minutes until everything is well combined and heated through.

5. **Serve:** Divide the pasta mixture among four plates. Garnish with grated Parmesan cheese, if desired. Serve warm.

Nutrients (per serving)

Calories: 350 kcal Carbohydrates: 45g Fiber: 5g

Protein: 25g Fat: 10g Sugar: 7g Sodium: 500mg

Calcium: 100mg

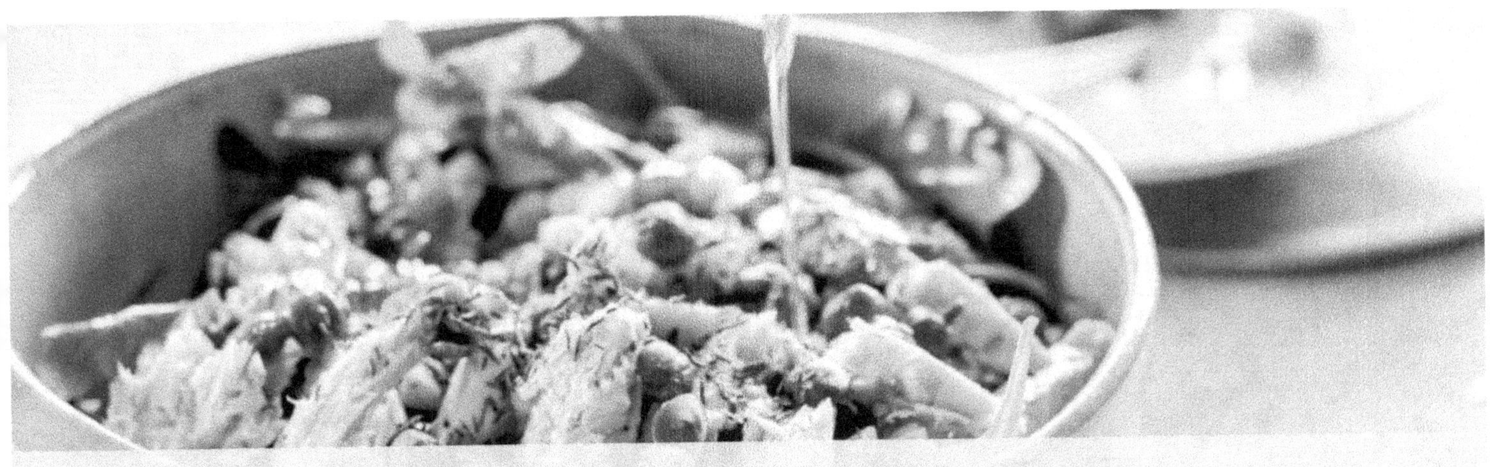

TUNA SALAD WITH OLIVE OIL

Tuna Salad with Olive Oil is a simple yet satisfying dish that blends the rich flavor of tuna with the subtle elegance of olive oil. Packed with protein and healthy fats, this salad is perfect for a quick lunch or a light dinner. The addition of fresh vegetables and a touch of lemon enhances the flavor while keeping the meal light and nutritious.

Serves		Preparation Time		Cooking Time	
4		10 minutes		0 minutes	

Ingredients:

- 2 cans (5 ounces each) tuna in water, drained
- 1/4 cup extra-virgin olive oil
- 1 tablespoon lemon juice
- 1 celery stalk, diced
- 1/2 red bell pepper, diced
- 1/4 cup red onion, finely chopped
- 1/4 cup chopped fresh parsley
- 1/2 teaspoon dried oregano
- 1/4 teaspoon black pepper
- 1/4 teaspoon salt
- 2 cups mixed salad greens (optional for serving)

Instructions:

1. **Prepare the Tuna:** In a large bowl, combine the drained tuna, diced celery, red bell pepper, red onion, and chopped parsley.
2. **Make the Dressing:** In a small bowl, whisk together the olive oil, lemon juice, dried oregano, black pepper, and salt.
3. **Combine and Toss:** Pour the dressing over the tuna mixture and gently toss until well combined and evenly coated.
4. **Serve:** Divide the tuna salad among four plates or bowls. Serve on a bed of mixed salad greens, if desired.

Nutrients (per serving)

Calories: 240 kcal Carbohydrates: 2g Fiber: 1g

Protein: 30g Fat: 12g Sugar: 1g Sodium: 300mg

Calcium: 40mg

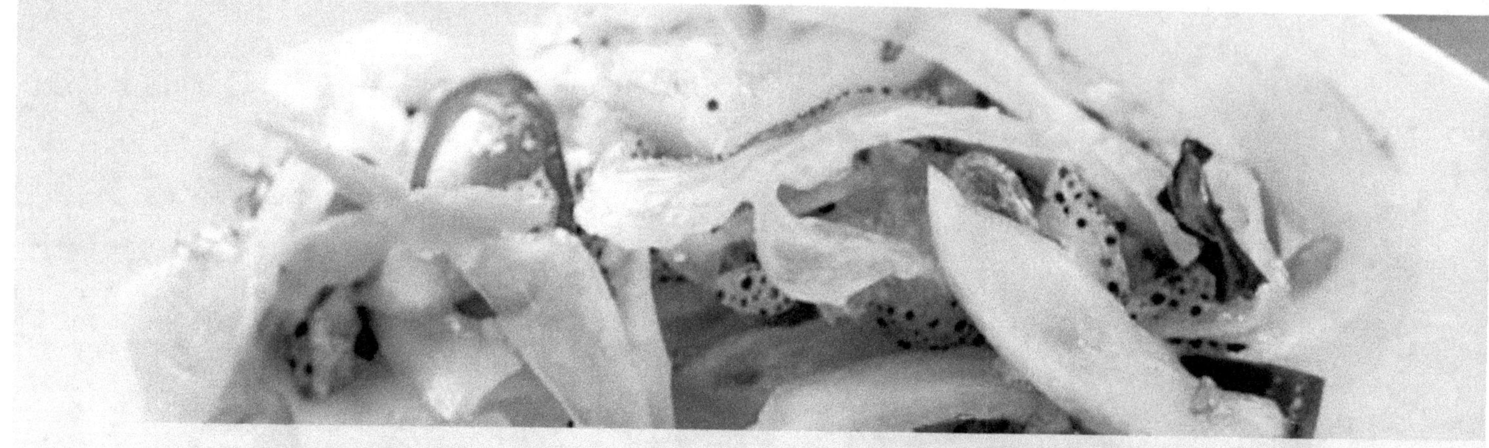

JELLYFISH SALAD WITH DRIED SHRIMP

Jellyfish Salad with Dried Shrimp is a unique and refreshing dish that combines the crisp, slightly crunchy texture of jellyfish with the savory depth of dried shrimp. This Asian-inspired salad is light, nutritious, and packed with bold flavors, making it an excellent choice for a healthy appetizer or a light meal.

Serves 	**Preparation Time** 	**Cooking Time** 
4	15 minutes	0 minutes

Ingredients:

1 cup dried jellyfish, rehydrated (see note)
1/4 cup dried shrimp, soaked and chopped
1/4 cup rice vinegar
2 tablespoons soy sauce
1 tablespoon sesame oil
1 tablespoon sucralose (optional for a touch of sweetness)
1 tablespoon grated ginger
1 garlic clove, minced
1/2 cucumber, julienned
1/2 red bell pepper, julienned
2 tablespoons chopped fresh cilantro
1 tablespoon sesame seeds (for garnish)

Instructions:

1. **Prepare the Jellyfish:** If using dried jellyfish, soak it in cold water for several hours or overnight until rehydrated. Drain and pat dry with paper towels.
2. **Prepare the Dried Shrimp:** Soak dried shrimp in warm water for 15 minutes to soften. Drain, then chop into small pieces.
3. **Make the Dressing:** In a small bowl, whisk together rice vinegar, soy sauce, sesame oil, sucralose (if using), grated ginger, and minced garlic.
4. **Combine Ingredients:** In a large bowl, mix the rehydrated jellyfish, chopped dried shrimp, julienned cucumber, and red bell pepper.
5. **Dress the Salad:** Pour the dressing over the salad mixture and toss gently to coat everything evenly.
6. **Garnish and Serve:** Sprinkle chopped fresh cilantro and sesame seeds on top before serving.

Nutrients (per serving)

Calories: 120 kcal Carbohydrates: 8g Fiber: 2g
Protein: 12g Fat: 5g Sugar: 2g Sodium: 700mg
Calcium: 60mg

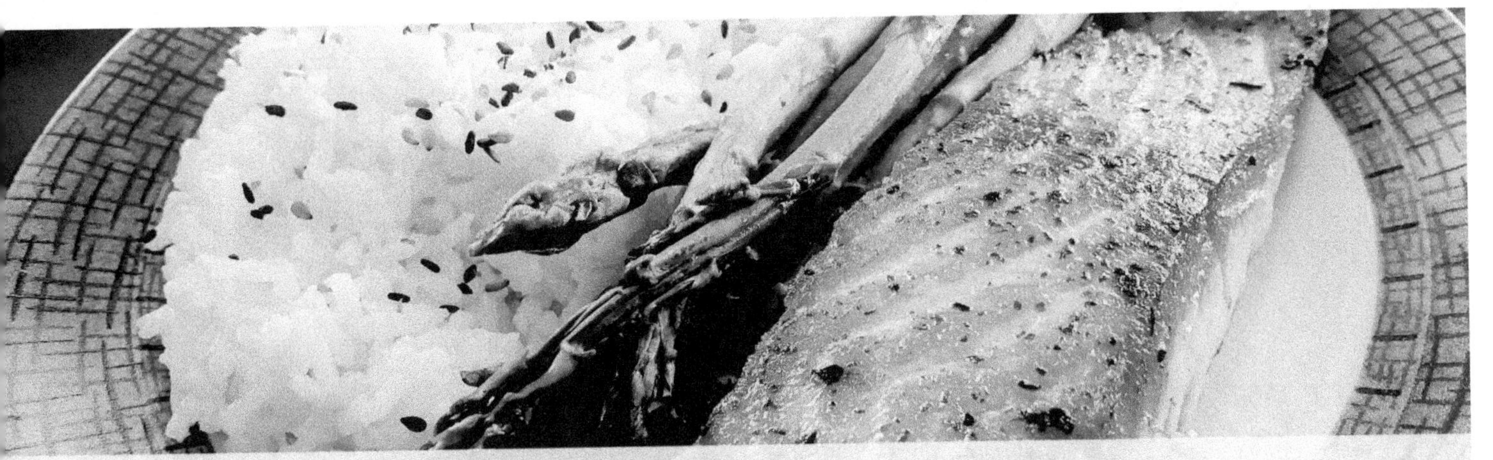

WHITE RICE WITH GRILLED SALMON

White Rice with Grilled Salmon is a classic, balanced meal that combines tender, flaky salmon with perfectly cooked white rice. This dish is simple yet satisfying, making it a go-to for a quick and healthy dinner. The grilled salmon provides a rich source of protein and omega-3 fatty acids, while the white rice offers a comforting and versatile base.

Serves	Preparation Time	Cooking Time
4	15 minutes	15 minutes

Ingredients:

4 salmon fillets (6 oz each)
1 tablespoon olive oil
1 tablespoon lemon juice
1 tablespoon sucralose (optional, for a touch of sweetness)
2 cloves garlic, minced
1 teaspoon dried dill
1 teaspoon dried parsley
Salt and pepper, to taste
2 cups white rice
4 cups water
1 tablespoon chopped fresh parsley (for garnish)
Lemon wedges (for serving)

Instructions:

1. **Prepare the Salmon:** In a small bowl, mix olive oil, lemon juice, sucralose (if using), minced garlic, dried dill, dried parsley, salt, and pepper. Brush the salmon fillets with the mixture on both sides.

2. **Grill the Salmon:** Preheat a grill or grill pan over medium-high heat. Place the salmon fillets on the grill and cook for about 4-5 minutes per side, or until the salmon flakes easily with a fork.

3. **Cook the Rice:** Rinse the white rice under cold water until the water runs clear. In a medium saucepan, bring 4 cups of water to a boil. Add the rice, reduce the heat to low, cover, and simmer for 15 minutes, or until the rice is tender and the water is absorbed. Fluff the rice with a fork and let it sit, covered, for 5 minutes.

4. **Serve:** Divide the cooked rice among four plates. Top each serving of rice with a grilled salmon fillet. Garnish with chopped fresh parsley and serve with lemon wedges on the side.

Nutrients (per serving)

Calories: 350 kcal Carbohydrates: 35g Fiber: 1g

Protein: 25g Fat: 15g Sugar: 1g Sodium: 120mg

Calcium: 25mg

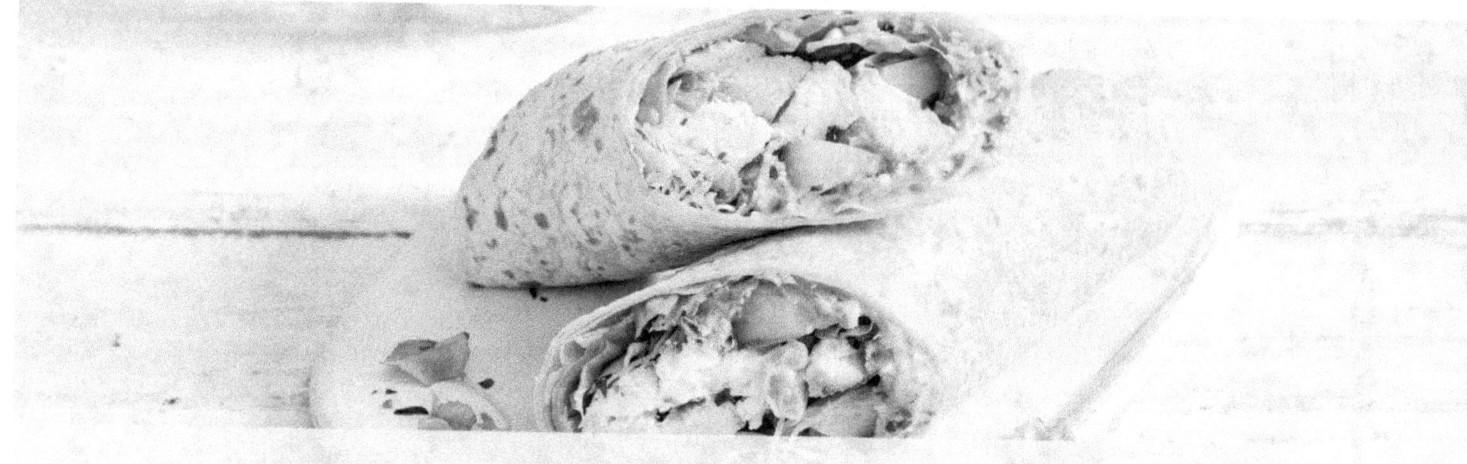

GRILLED CHICKEN WRAP WITH GREENS

The Grilled Chicken Wrap with Greens is a delicious and nutritious meal that combines tender grilled chicken with fresh greens and a whole grain wrap. This wrap is perfect for a quick lunch or dinner, offering a balanced blend of protein, fiber, and vitamins. The light yet flavorful dressing enhances the freshness of the greens, making each bite satisfying and healthy.

Serves 	Preparation Time 	Cooking Time 
4	10 minutes	10 minutes

Ingredients:

2 boneless, skinless chicken breasts
1 tablespoon olive oil
1 teaspoon paprika
1 teaspoon garlic powder
1 teaspoon dried oregano
Salt and pepper, to taste
4 whole grain wraps
2 cups mixed greens (such as spinach, arugula, and romaine)
1 cup cherry tomatoes, halved
1 cucumber, sliced
1/2 red onion, thinly sliced
1/4 cup low-fat Greek yogurt (for dressing)
1 tablespoon lemon juice
1 teaspoon honey or sucralose (optional, for sweetness)
1 teaspoon Dijon mustard
1 tablespoon chopped fresh basil (for garnish)

Instructions:

1. **Prepare the Chicken:** Preheat a grill or grill pan over medium-high heat. Rub the chicken breasts with olive oil, paprika, garlic powder, dried oregano, salt, and pepper. Grill the chicken for about 5-7 minutes per side, or until fully cooked and the internal temperature reaches 165°F (74°C). Remove from the grill and let rest for a few minutes before slicing into strips.
2. **Prepare the Wraps:** In a small bowl, mix Greek yogurt, lemon juice, honey or sucralose (if using), and Dijon mustard to make the dressing. Adjust seasoning with salt and pepper to taste. Spread a thin layer of the dressing on each whole grain wrap.
3. **Assemble the Wraps:** On each wrap, layer the mixed greens, cherry tomatoes, cucumber slices, and red onion. Top with sliced grilled chicken. Sprinkle with chopped fresh basil.
4. **Roll and Serve:** Carefully roll up each wrap, tucking in the sides as you go to keep the fillings inside. Slice the wraps in half diagonally and serve immediately.

Nutrients (per serving)

Calories: 350 kcal Carbohydrates: 30g Fiber: 5g
Protein: 30g Fat: 10g Sugar: 4g Sodium: 200mg
Calcium: 50mg

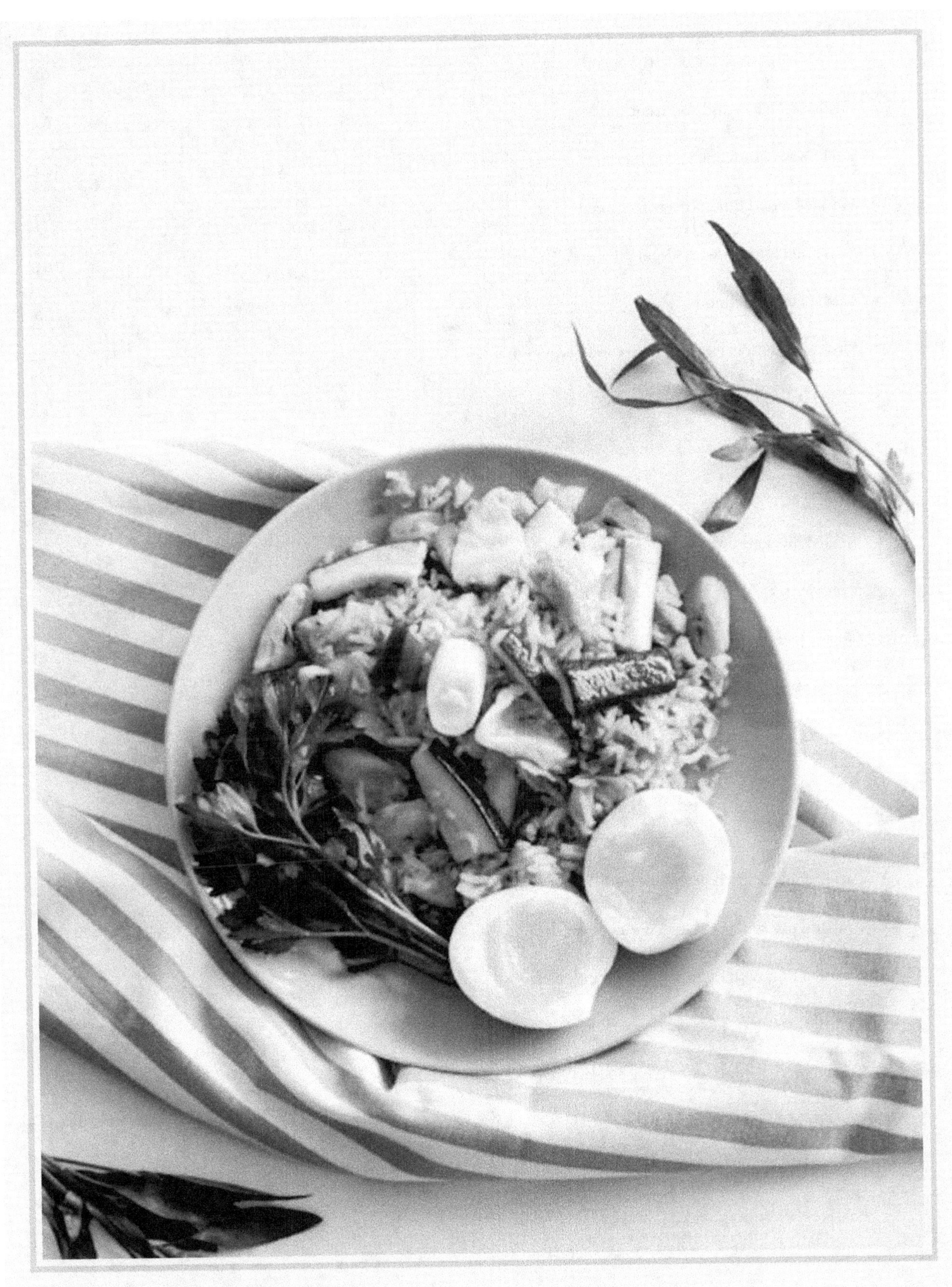

TABLE OF CONTENTS

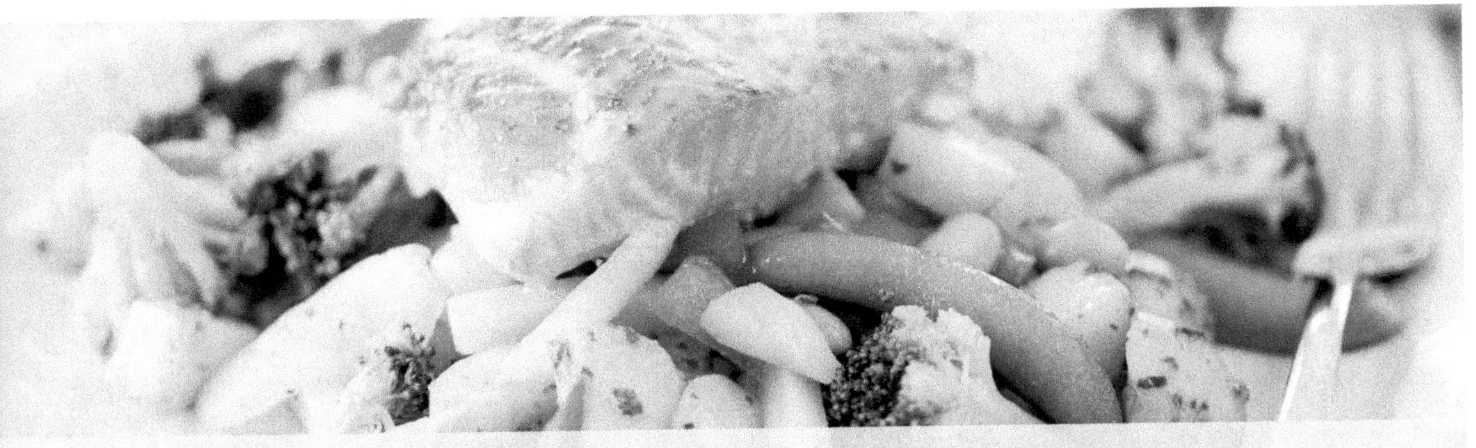

BAKED SALMON WITH ROASTED VEGETABLES

Baked Salmon with Roasted Vegetables is a wholesome and flavorful dish that combines tender, oven-baked salmon with a medley of roasted vegetables. This meal is packed with nutrients and omega-3 fatty acids from the salmon and provides a satisfying, balanced dinner option. The roasted vegetables add a delicious caramelized flavor and a variety of textures to complement the salmon.

Serves	Preparation Time	Cooking Time
4	15 minutes	30 minute

Ingredients:

4 salmon fillets (about 6 oz each)

2 tablespoons olive oil

1 teaspoon garlic powder

1 teaspoon dried thyme

1 teaspoon paprika

Salt and pepper, to taste

2 cups baby carrots

1 red bell pepper, chopped

1 zucchini, sliced

1 red onion, chopped

1 tablespoon fresh lemon juice

1 tablespoon chopped fresh parsley (for garnish)

Instructions:

1. **Preheat Oven:** Preheat your oven to 400°F (200°C).
2. **Prepare the Salmon:** Place the salmon fillets on a baking sheet lined with parchment paper or aluminum foil. Brush the salmon with 1 tablespoon of olive oil. Sprinkle garlic powder, dried thyme, paprika, salt, and pepper evenly over the salmon fillets.
3. **Prepare the Vegetables:** In a large bowl, toss the baby carrots, red bell pepper, zucchini, and red onion with the remaining 1 tablespoon of olive oil. Season the vegetables with salt and pepper to taste.
4. **Bake:** Spread the seasoned vegetables around the salmon fillets on the baking sheet. Bake in the preheated oven for about 20-25 minutes, or until the salmon is cooked through and flakes easily with a fork. The vegetables should be tender and slightly caramelized.
5. **Finish and Serve:** Drizzle fresh lemon juice over the salmon fillets and vegetables. Garnish with chopped fresh parsley. Serve immediately.

Nutrients (per serving)

Calories: 350 kcal Carbohydrates: 20g Fiber: 5g

Protein: 30g Fat: 18g Sugar: 8g Sodium: 200mg

Calcium: 60mg

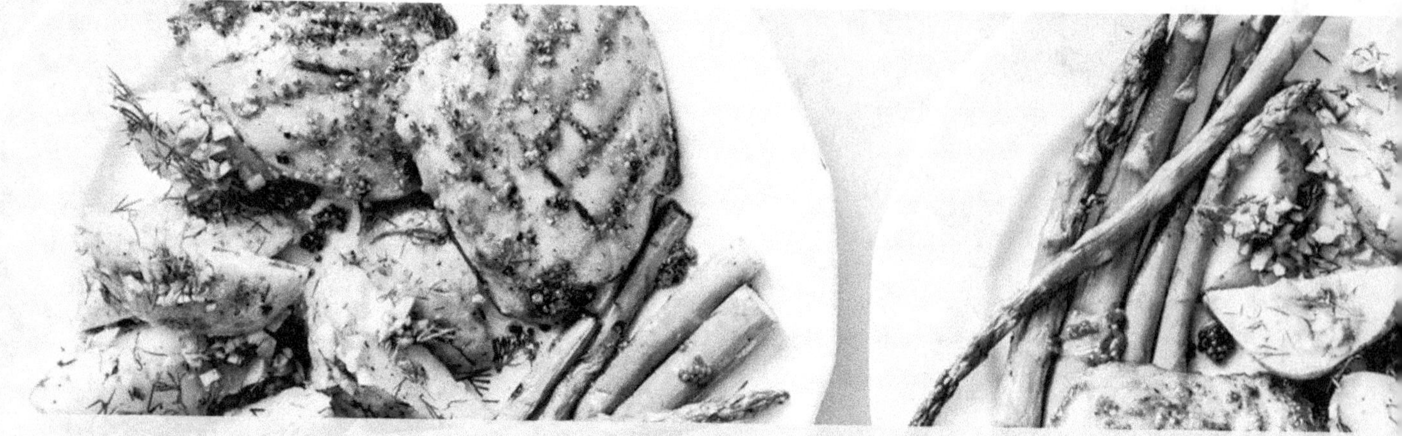

GRILLED CHICKEN AND ASPARAGUS

Grilled Chicken and Asparagus is a healthy, light meal that brings together juicy, marinated chicken breasts and tender, charred asparagus. This dish is simple yet flavorful, offering a great balance of protein and vegetables. The grilling process imparts a delicious smoky flavor to both the chicken and asparagus, making it a perfect option for a nutritious lunch or dinner.

Serves		**Preparation Time**		**Cooking Time**	
4		15 minutes		15 minute	

Ingredients:

4 boneless, skinless chicken breasts (about 6 oz each)

1 pound (450g) asparagus spears, trimmed

2 tablespoons olive oil

1 tablespoon lemon juice

1 teaspoon garlic powder

1 teaspoon dried oregano

1 teaspoon paprika

Salt and pepper, to taste

Lemon wedges (for serving)

Fresh parsley, chopped (for garnish)

Instructions:

1. **Prepare the Marinade:** In a small bowl, mix together olive oil, lemon juice, garlic powder, dried oregano, paprika, salt, and pepper.
2. **Marinate the Chicken:** Place the chicken breasts in a resealable plastic bag or shallow dish.Pour the marinade over the chicken and toss to coat evenly. Let the chicken marinate in the refrigerator for at least 30 minutes, or up to 4 hours for more flavor.
3. **Preheat the Grill:** Preheat your grill to medium-high heat.
4. **Grill the Chicken and Asparagus:** Remove the chicken breasts from the marinade and discard any excess marinade.Place the chicken on the grill and cook for 6-7 minutes per side, or until the internal temperature reaches 165°F (74°C) and the chicken is no longer pink in the center.While the chicken is grilling, toss the asparagus with a small amount of olive oil, salt, and pepper.Grill the asparagus for about 4-5 minutes, turning occasionally, until tender and slightly charred.
5. **Serve:** Remove the chicken and asparagus from the grill.Slice the chicken breasts and arrange them on a serving platter alongside the grilled asparagus.Garnish with fresh parsley and serve with lemon wedges.

Nutrients (per serving)

Calories: 300 kcal Carbohydrates: 8g Fiber: 3g

Protein: 40g Fat: 12g Sugar: 3g Sodium: 200mg

Calcium: 50mg

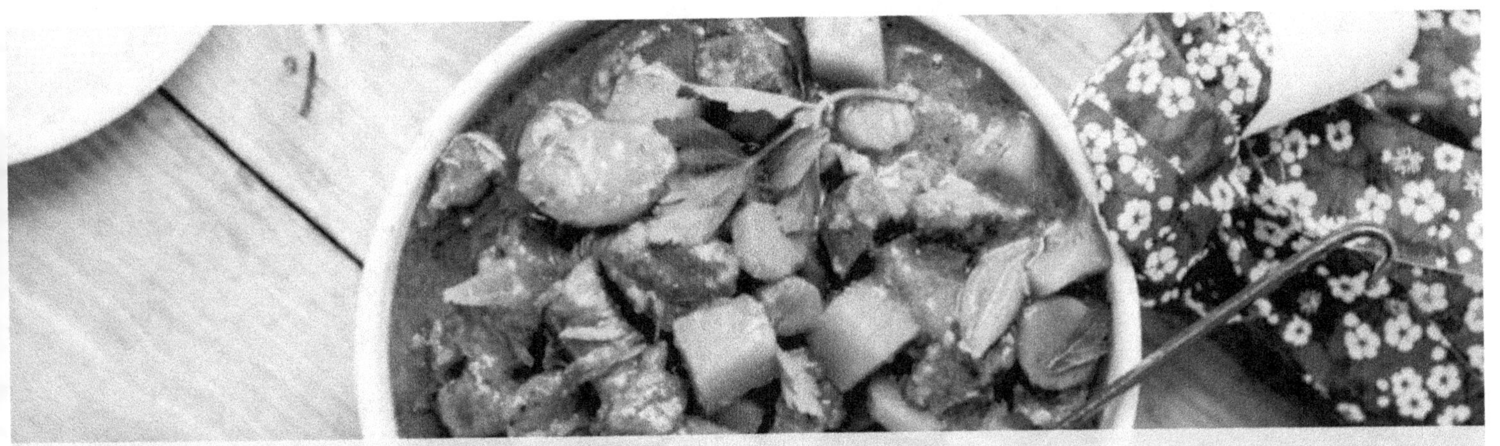

BEEF STEW WITH ROOT VEGETABLES

Beef Stew with Root Vegetables is a hearty and comforting dish that's perfect for a satisfying meal. This stew features tender chunks of beef simmered with a medley of root vegetables in a rich, savory broth. It's an ideal choice for a nourishing dinner, especially on cooler days, and provides a balanced combination of protein and vegetables.

Serves		Preparation Time		Cooking Time	
4		20 minutes		90 minute	

Ingredients:

1.5 pounds (680g) beef chuck, cut into 1-inch cubes
2 tablespoons olive oil
1 large onion, diced
3 cloves garlic, minced
4 cups beef broth (low-sodium)
1 cup water
1 tablespoon tomato paste
1 tablespoon Worcestershire sauce
1 teaspoon dried thyme
1 teaspoon dried rosemary
1 bay leaf
3 medium carrots, peeled and cut into chunks
2 medium potatoes, peeled and cut into chunks
1 parsnip, peeled and cut into chunks
1 cup frozen peas
Salt and pepper, to taste
Fresh parsley, chopped (for garnish)

Instructions:

1. **Brown the Beef:** Heat olive oil in a large pot or Dutch oven over medium-high heat.Add the beef cubes and cook until browned on all sides, about 5-7 minutes. Work in batches if necessary to avoid overcrowding the pot. Remove the browned beef and set aside.
2. **Sauté the Vegetables:** In the same pot, add diced onion and cook until softened, about 3-4 minutes.Add minced garlic and cook for another 1 minute.
3. **Prepare the Stew Base:** Return the browned beef to the pot.Stir in tomato paste and cook for 1 minute.Pour in beef broth and water, scraping the bottom of the pot to release any browned bits.Add Worcestershire sauce, dried thyme, dried rosemary, and bay leaf. Stir well to combine.
4. **Simmer the Stew:** Bring the stew to a boil, then reduce the heat to low.
5. Cover and let simmer for 1 hour, or until the beef is tender.
6. **Add the Root Vegetables:** After 1 hour, add carrots, potatoes, and parsnips to the stew.Continue to simmer, covered, for an additional 30 minutes, or until the vegetables are tender.
7. **Finish the Stew:** Stir in frozen peas and cook for another 5 minutes.Season with salt and pepper to taste.Remove the bay leaf.
8. **Serve:** Ladle the stew into bowls and garnish with chopped fresh parsley.

Nutrients (per serving)

Calories: 350 kcal Carbohydrates: 30g Fiber: 7g
Protein: 30g Fat: 14g Sugar: 8g Sodium: 600mg
Calcium: 80mg

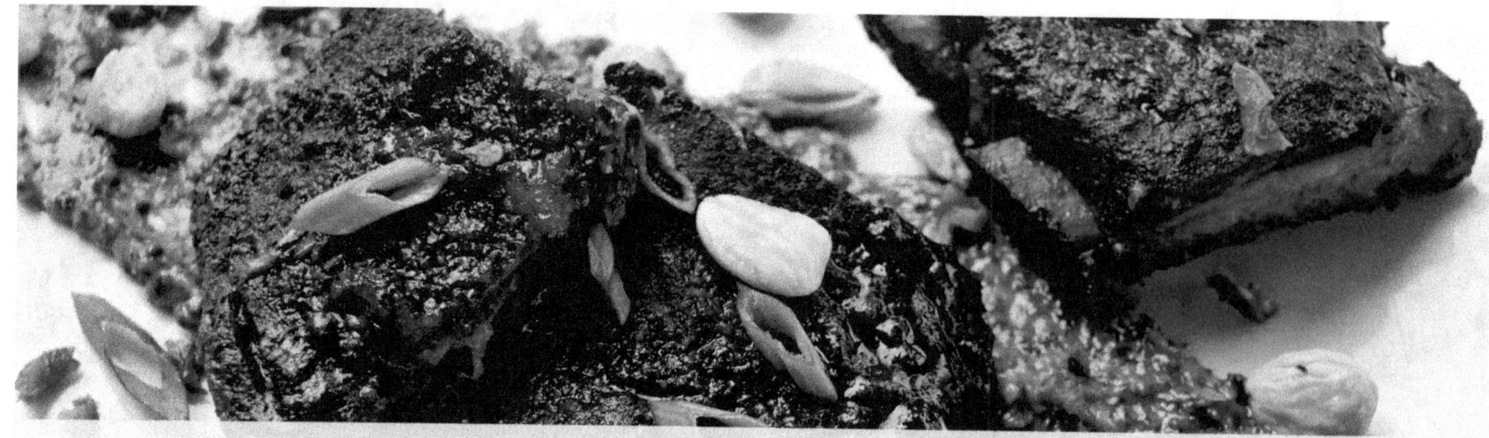

HONEY-GLAZED PORK RIBS WITH GREENS

Honey-Glazed Pork Ribs with Greens is a delectable dish that combines succulent pork ribs with a sweet and savory honey glaze. The glaze caramelizes during cooking, creating a deliciously sticky and flavorful coating. Paired with a side of fresh, sautéed greens, this meal is both satisfying and balanced, perfect for a special dinner or a weekend treat.

Serves		Preparation Time		Cooking Time	
4		20 minutes		75 minutes	

Ingredients:

For the Pork Ribs:

2 pounds (900g) pork ribs

1/4 cup honey

1/4 cup soy sauce (low-sodium)

2 tablespoons apple cider vinegar

2 tablespoons hoisin sauce

2 cloves garlic, minced

1 teaspoon ginger, grated

1 teaspoon ground black pepper

1/2 teaspoon salt

1 tablespoon olive oil

For the Greens:

1 tablespoon olive oil

4 cups mixed greens (such as spinach, kale, and Swiss chard)

2 cloves garlic, minced

1/4 teaspoon red pepper flakes (optional)

Salt and pepper, to taste

Instructions:

1. **Prepare the Pork Ribs:** Preheat your oven to 300°F (150°C).In a bowl, combine honey, soy sauce, apple cider vinegar, hoisin sauce, minced garlic, grated ginger, black pepper, and salt. Stir until well mixed.Place the pork ribs on a large baking sheet lined with aluminum foil. Brush both sides of the ribs with olive oil.Generously brush the honey glaze over the ribs, coating them well.

2. **Cook the Ribs:** Cover the baking sheet with aluminum foil.Bake in the preheated oven for 1 hour.After 1 hour, remove the foil and brush the ribs with more honey glaze.Return to the oven and bake for an additional 15-20 minutes, or until the ribs are tender and the glaze has caramelized.

3. **Prepare the Greens:** While the ribs are finishing, heat olive oil in a large skillet over medium heat.Add minced garlic and cook for 1 minute until fragrant.Add the mixed greens and cook, stirring frequently, until wilted, about 3-4 minutes.If using, add red pepper flakes for a bit of heat.Season with salt and pepper to taste.

4. **Serve:** Slice the honey-glazed ribs between the bones.Serve the ribs alongside the sautéed greens.

Nutrients (per serving)

Calories: 450 kcal Carbohydrates: 20g Fiber: 3g

Protein: 35g Fat: 25g Sugar: 15g Sodium: 800mg

Calcium: 100mg

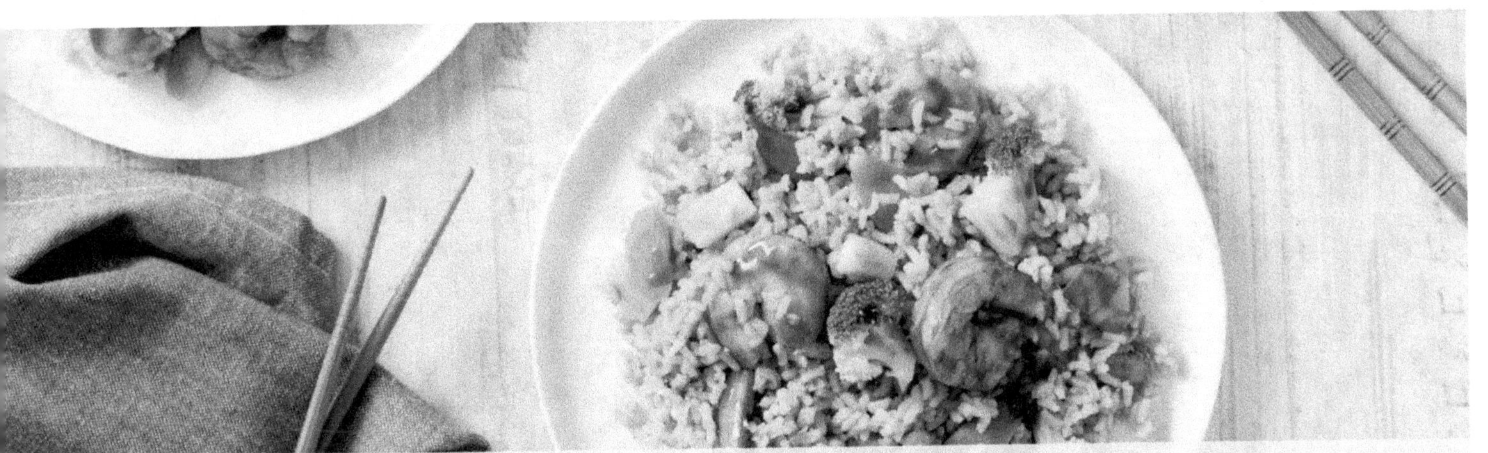

STIR-FRIED SHRIMP WITH VEGETABLES AND BROWN RICE

Stir-Fried Shrimp with Vegetables and Brown Rice is a quick and healthy dish that's packed with flavor and nutrients. The shrimp are lightly seasoned and stir-fried with a colorful mix of vegetables, served over wholesome brown rice. This meal is perfect for a busy weeknight or a nutritious lunch, offering a balanced combination of protein, fiber, and essential vitamins.

Serves	**Preparation Time**	**Cooking Time**
4	15 minutes	20 minutes

Ingredients:

For the Stir-Fry:

1 pound (450g) large shrimp, peeled and deveined

2 tablespoons olive oil

1 red bell pepper, sliced

1 yellow bell pepper, sliced

1 cup broccoli florets

1 cup snap peas

2 cloves garlic, minced

1 tablespoon ginger, minced

3 tablespoons low-sodium soy sauce

1 tablespoon honey

1 tablespoon rice vinegar

1 teaspoon sesame oil

1 tablespoon cornstarch mixed with 2 tablespoons water (optional, for thickening)

Salt and pepper, to taste

For the Brown Rice:

1 cup brown rice

2 cups water

1/4 teaspoon salt

Instructions:

1. **Prepare the Brown Rice:** Rinse the brown rice under cold water until the water runs clear.In a medium saucepan, bring 2 cups of water and 1/4 teaspoon salt to a boil.Add the rinsed rice, reduce heat to low, and cover.Simmer for 45-50 minutes, or until the rice is tender and the water is absorbed. Fluff with a fork and keep warm.

2. **Cook the Stir-Fry:** Heat olive oil in a large skillet or wok over medium-high heat.Add minced garlic and ginger, and cook for 1 minute until fragrant.Add the shrimp to the skillet and cook for 2-3 minutes on each side, or until they turn pink and opaque. Remove shrimp from the skillet and set aside.In the same skillet, add the bell peppers, broccoli, and snap peas. Stir-fry for 5-6 minutes, or until the vegetables are tender-crisp.Return the shrimp to the skillet.In a small bowl, mix together the soy sauce, honey, rice vinegar, and sesame oil. Pour the sauce over the shrimp and vegetables.Stir well to coat everything with the sauce. If you prefer a thicker sauce, add the cornstarch mixture and cook for an additional 1-2 minutes until the sauce has thickened.Season with salt and pepper to taste.

3. **Serve:** Divide the cooked brown rice among four plates.Top each plate with the stir-fried shrimp and vegetables.

Nutrients (per serving)

Calories: 350 kcal Carbohydrates: 45g Fiber: 6g

Protein: 25g Fat: 10g Sugar: 10g Sodium: 800mg

Calcium: 80mg

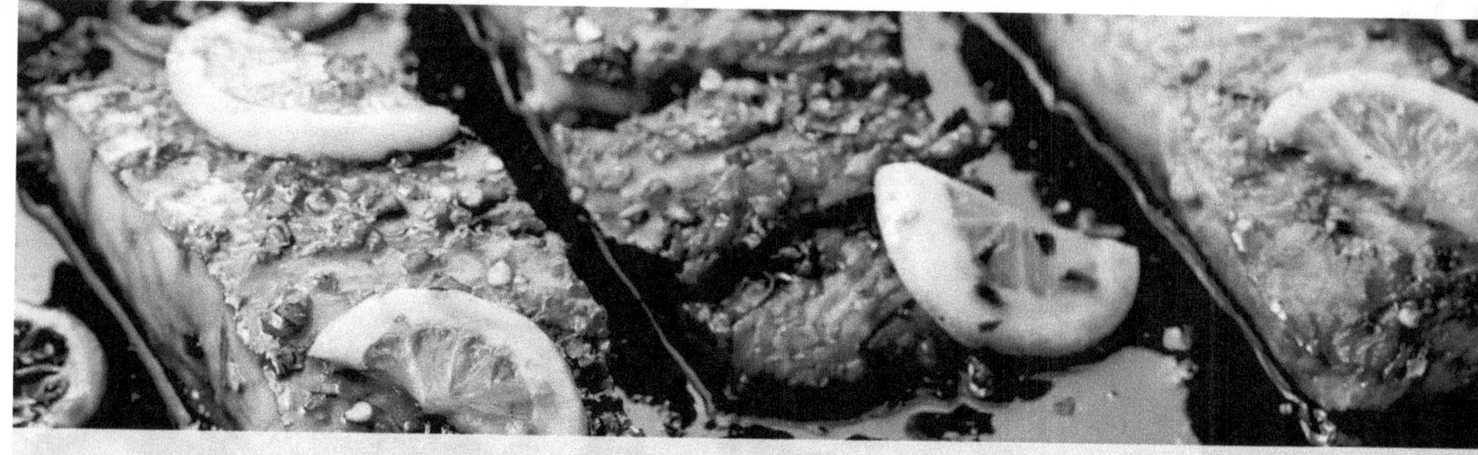

GARLIC HONEY SALMON

Garlic Honey Salmon is a delicious and easy-to-make dish that combines the rich flavors of garlic and honey with succulent salmon fillets. This recipe is perfect for a quick weeknight dinner or a special occasion, offering a sweet and savory glaze that enhances the natural flavors of the fish. Served with your choice of side dishes, this meal is sure to please everyone at the table.

Serves	Preparation Time	Cooking Time
4	10 minutes	15 minutes

Ingredients:

4 salmon fillets (about 6 ounces each)
2 tablespoons olive oil
3 cloves garlic, minced
1/4 cup honey
2 tablespoons soy sauce (low-sodium)
1 tablespoon Dijon mustard
1 tablespoon lemon juice
1 teaspoon dried thyme or rosemary
Salt and pepper, to taste
Lemon wedges, for garnish (optional)
Fresh parsley, chopped, for garnish (optional)

Instructions:

1. **Prepare the Oven:** Preheat your oven to 400°F (200°C). Line a baking sheet with parchment paper or lightly grease it.
2. **Make the Glaze:** In a small saucepan, heat the olive oil over medium heat.Add the minced garlic and sauté for 1 minute until fragrant, but not browned.Stir in the honey, soy sauce, Dijon mustard, lemon juice, and dried thyme (or rosemary).Cook for 2-3 minutes, stirring occasionally, until the glaze slightly thickens. Remove from heat.
3. **Prepare the Salmon:** Season the salmon fillets with salt and pepper.Place the salmon fillets on the prepared baking sheet.
4. **Glaze the Salmon:** Brush the garlic honey glaze generously over each salmon fillet.Reserve some of the glaze for drizzling over the salmon after baking, if desired.
5. **Bake the Salmon:** Bake the salmon in the preheated oven for 12-15 minutes, or until the salmon is cooked through and flakes easily with a fork. The internal temperature should reach 145°F (63°C).
6. **Serve:** Transfer the salmon fillets to serving plates.Drizzle with the reserved glaze, if using.Garnish with lemon wedges and chopped parsley, if desired.

Nutrients (per serving)

Calories: 280 kcal Carbohydrates: 22g Fiber: 0g
Protein: 26g Fat: 14g Sugar: 18g Sodium: 600mg
Calcium: 30mg

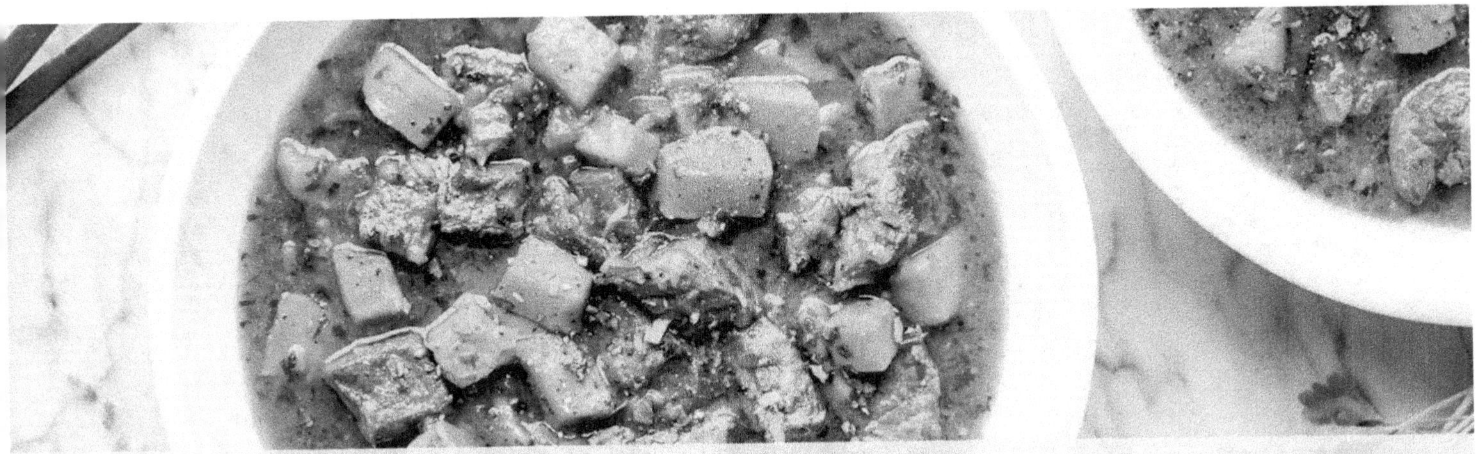

SLOW-COOKED BEEF WITH CARROTS AND SWEET POTATOES

Slow-Cooked Beef with Carrots and Sweet Potatoes is a comforting and hearty dish that's perfect for a cozy meal. The beef becomes incredibly tender as it simmers in a savory broth, while the carrots and sweet potatoes absorb the rich flavors of the slow cooker. This recipe is ideal for busy days when you want a nutritious and delicious dinner with minimal effort.

Serves		**Preparation Time**		**Cooking Time**	
4		15 minutes		8 hours	

Ingredients:

- 2 pounds beef chuck roast, cut into 1-inch cubes
- 4 medium carrots, peeled and sliced
- 2 medium sweet potatoes, peeled and cubed
- 1 onion, chopped
- 3 cloves garlic, minced
- 2 cups beef broth (low-sodium)
- 1/2 cup red wine (optional, or additional beef broth)
- 2 tablespoons tomato paste
- 1 tablespoon Worcestershire sauce
- 1 teaspoon dried thyme
- 1 teaspoon dried rosemary
- Salt and pepper, to taste
- 2 tablespoons olive oil

Instructions:

1. **Prepare the Beef:** Season the beef cubes with salt and pepper. Heat olive oil in a large skillet over medium-high heat. Brown the beef cubes in batches, about 3-4 minutes per side, until browned. Transfer to the slow cooker.
2. **Prepare the Vegetables:** In the same skillet, sauté the chopped onion and minced garlic until softened, about 3 minutes. Add the tomato paste and cook for another 1 minute. Transfer the onion mixture to the slow cooker.
3. **Combine Ingredients:** Add the sliced carrots and cubed sweet potatoes to the slow cooker. Pour in the beef broth and red wine (if using). Stir in Worcestershire sauce, dried thyme, and dried rosemary.
4. **Slow Cook:** Cover the slow cooker and cook on low for 8 hours, or until the beef is tender and the vegetables are cooked through.
5. **Serve:** Taste and adjust seasoning with additional salt and pepper if needed. Serve hot, garnished with fresh parsley if desired.

Nutrients (per serving)

Calories: 370 kcal Carbohydrates: 30g Fiber: 6g

Protein: 30g Fat: 15g Sugar: 8g Sodium: 600mg

Calcium: 60mg

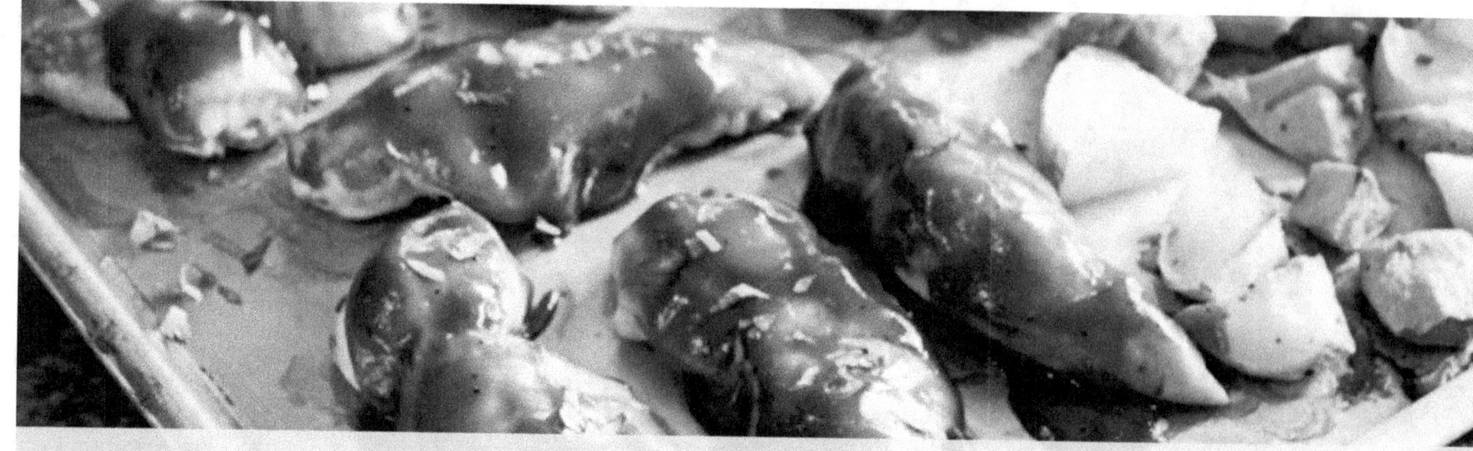

BBQ GRILLED CHICKEN WITH ROASTED POTATOES

BBQ Grilled Chicken with Roasted Potatoes is a delightful dish that combines smoky, grilled chicken with crispy roasted potatoes. This recipe is perfect for a summer barbecue or a casual family dinner. The chicken is marinated in a flavorful BBQ sauce, then grilled to perfection, while the potatoes are seasoned and roasted until golden brown.

Serves	Preparation Time	Cooking Time
 4	20 minutes	 30 minutes

Ingredients:

For the BBQ Grilled Chicken:

4 boneless, skinless chicken breasts

1 cup BBQ sauce (store-bought or homemade)

2 tablespoons olive oil

1 teaspoon garlic powder

1 teaspoon paprika

1/2 teaspoon onion powder

Salt and pepper, to taste

For the Roasted Potatoes:

1 pound baby potatoes, halved

2 tablespoons olive oil

1 teaspoon dried rosemary

1 teaspoon dried thyme

1/2 teaspoon garlic powder

Salt and pepper, to taste

Instructions:

1. **Marinate the Chicken:** In a bowl, mix together the BBQ sauce, olive oil, garlic powder, paprika, onion powder, salt, and pepper.Coat the chicken breasts with the BBQ sauce mixture.Cover and refrigerate for at least 1 hour, or overnight for best results.

2. **Prepare the Potatoes:** Preheat the oven to 400°F (200°C).In a large bowl, toss the halved baby potatoes with olive oil, dried rosemary, dried thyme, garlic powder, salt, and pepper.Spread the potatoes in a single layer on a baking sheet.

3. **Roast the Potatoes:** Roast the potatoes in the preheated oven for 25-30 minutes, or until golden brown and crispy, tossing halfway through.

4. **Grill the Chicken:** Preheat the grill to medium-high heat.Remove the chicken breasts from the marinade and discard the excess marinade.Grill the chicken for 6-8 minutes per side, or until the internal temperature reaches 165°F (74°C) and the chicken is cooked through.Let the chicken rest for a few minutes before serving.

5. **Serve:** Serve the BBQ grilled chicken alongside the roasted potatoes. Garnish with fresh herbs if desired.

Nutrients (per serving)

Calories: 430 kcal Carbohydrates: 38g Fiber: 5g

Protein: 35g Fat: 18g Sugar: 12g Sodium: 800mg

Calcium: 50mg

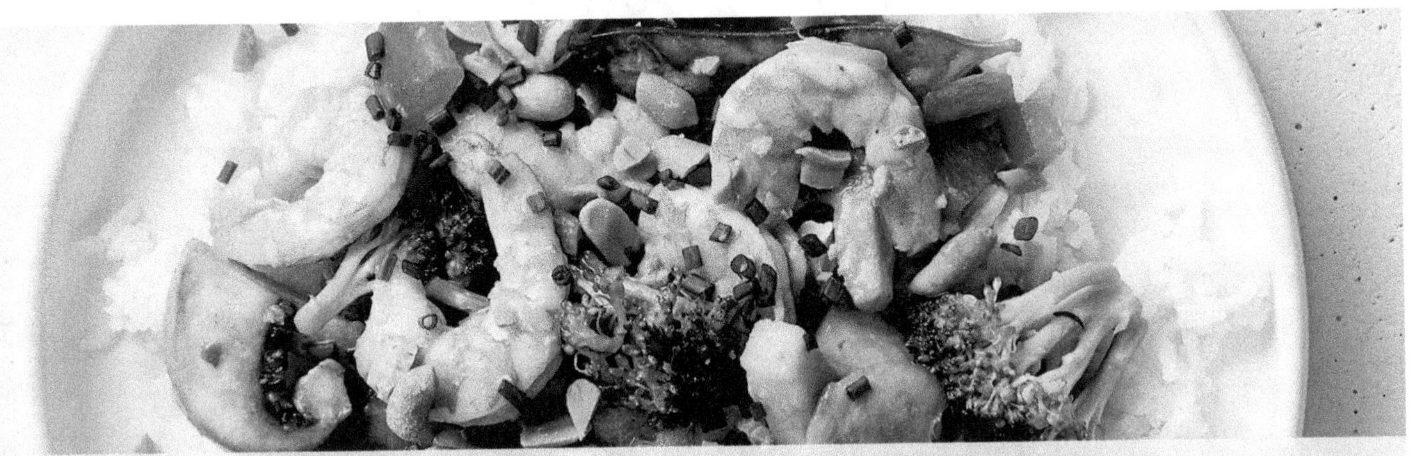

STEAMED SHRIMP WITH LEMONGRASS AND BROWN RICE

Steamed Shrimp with Lemongrass and Brown Rice is a fresh and healthy dish that features succulent shrimp steamed with aromatic lemongrass, paired with nutty brown rice. This recipe highlights the vibrant flavors of lemongrass and is perfect for a light and nutritious meal. It's easy to prepare and ideal for a quick dinner or a meal prep option.

Serves		Preparation Time		Cooking Time	
4		15 minutes		20 minutes	

Ingredients:

For the Steamed Shrimp:

1 pound large shrimp, peeled and deveined

2 stalks lemongrass, trimmed and cut into 2-inch pieces

3 cloves garlic, minced

1 tablespoon soy sauce (or tamari for gluten-free)

1 teaspoon fish sauce (optional)

1 tablespoon fresh lime juice

1 teaspoon ginger, grated

Salt and pepper, to taste

For the Brown Rice:

1 cup brown rice

2 cups water

1/2 teaspoon salt

Instructions:

1. **Prepare the Brown Rice:** Rinse the brown rice under cold water until the water runs clear.In a medium saucepan, combine the rice, water, and salt.Bring to a boil, then reduce heat to low, cover, and simmer for 40-45 minutes, or until the rice is tender and the water is absorbed.Remove from heat and let it sit, covered, for 5 minutes. Fluff with a fork before serving.

2. **Prepare the Steamed Shrimp:** In a bowl, combine the shrimp with soy sauce, fish sauce (if using), lime juice, garlic, ginger, salt, and pepper. Toss to coat evenly.Place lemongrass pieces in a steamer basket or a heatproof dish that fits into a steamer.Arrange the shrimp on top of the lemongrass.Steam the shrimp over boiling water for 5-7 minutes, or until the shrimp are pink and opaque. Be careful not to overcook them.

3. **Serve:** Divide the brown rice among four plates.Top with the steamed shrimp.Garnish with additional lime wedges or fresh herbs if desired.

Nutrients (per serving)

Calories: 350 kcal Carbohydrates: 40g Fiber: 4g

Protein: 25g Fat: 6g Sugar: 2g Sodium: 700mg

Calcium: 40mg

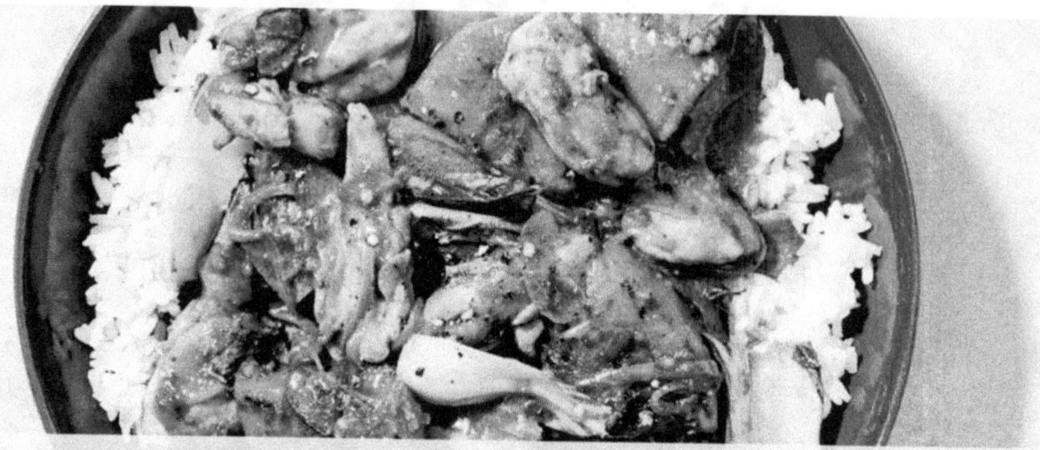

STIR-FRIED CHICKEN WITH LEMONGRASS AND BOK CHOY

Stir-Fried Chicken with Lemongrass and Bok Choy is a flavorful and vibrant dish that combines tender chicken with the aromatic essence of lemongrass and the crisp freshness of bok choy. This quick and easy stir-fry is perfect for a healthy weeknight dinner, packed with nutrients and delicious flavors.

Serves	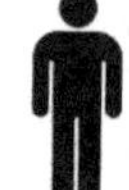 Preparation Time	 Cooking Time	
4	15 minutes	10 minutes	

Ingredients:

1 pound chicken breast or thighs, thinly sliced

2 tablespoons vegetable oil

2 stalks lemongrass, trimmed and finely chopped

3 cloves garlic, minced

1 tablespoon fresh ginger, minced

1 red bell pepper, sliced

2 cups bok choy, chopped

1 tablespoon soy sauce (or tamari for gluten-free)

1 tablespoon fish sauce (optional)

1 teaspoon honey or sucralose (optional for sweetness)

1 tablespoon rice vinegar

1/2 teaspoon red pepper flakes (optional for heat)

Salt and pepper, to taste

Fresh cilantro or green onions for garnish (optional)

Instructions:

1. **Prepare the Ingredients:** Slice the chicken thinly and chop the lemongrass finely.Mince the garlic and ginger.Slice the red bell pepper and chop the bok choy.

2. **Cook the Chicken:** Heat vegetable oil in a large skillet or wok over medium-high heat.Add the chopped lemongrass, garlic, and ginger, and sauté for 1-2 minutes until fragrant.Add the sliced chicken to the skillet. Stir-fry for 5-6 minutes, or until the chicken is cooked through and no longer pink.

3. **Add Vegetables and Seasonings:** Add the sliced red bell pepper and chopped bok choy to the skillet. Stir-fry for an additional 3-4 minutes until the vegetables are tender-crisp.Stir in the soy sauce, fish sauce (if using), honey or sucralose (if using), and rice vinegar. Mix well to coat the chicken and vegetables.Add red pepper flakes if desired, and season with salt and pepper to taste.

4. **Serve:** Garnish with fresh cilantro or green onions if desired.Serve the stir-fry over steamed rice or noodles if preferred.

Nutrients (per serving)

Calories: 280 kcal Carbohydrates: 15g Fiber: 3g

Protein: 25g Fat: 14g Sugar: 7g Sodium: 850mg

Calcium: 60mg

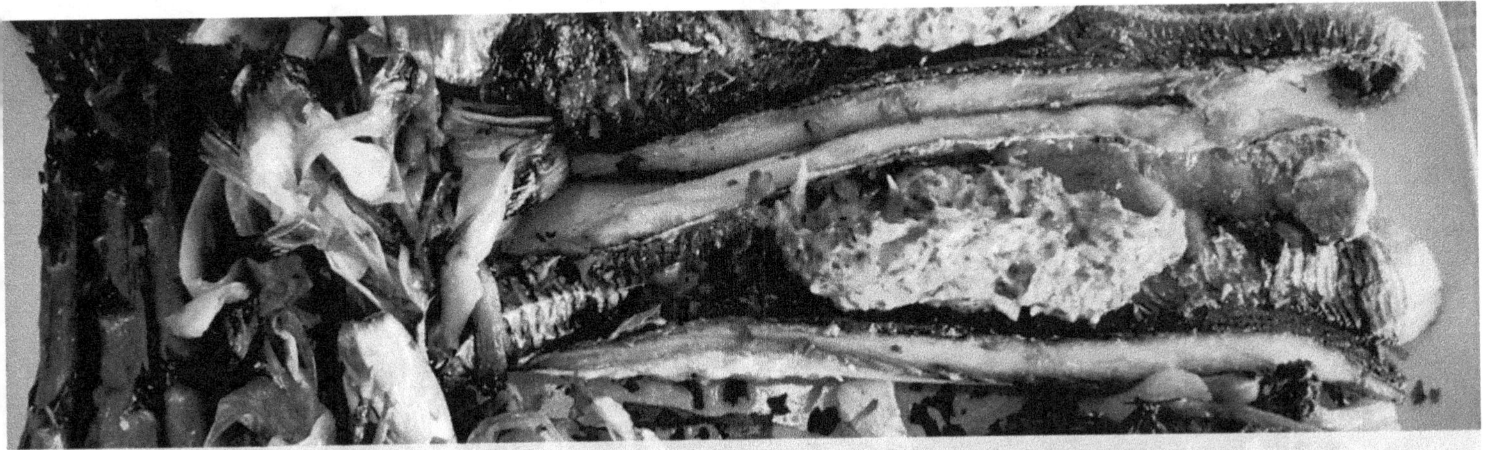

GRILLED MACKEREL WITH ROASTED VEGETABLES

Grilled Mackerel with Roasted Vegetables is a wholesome and satisfying dish that combines the rich, savory flavor of mackerel with a medley of tender, roasted vegetables. This recipe is not only nutritious but also easy to prepare, making it an excellent choice for a balanced weeknight dinner.

Serves	Preparation Time	Cooking Time
4	15 minutes	30 minutes

Ingredients:

4 mackerel fillets (about 6 ounces each)

2 tablespoons olive oil

1 teaspoon dried thyme

1 teaspoon paprika

1 teaspoon garlic powder

1 lemon, sliced

Salt and pepper, to taste

2 cups baby potatoes, halved

1 red bell pepper, chopped

1 zucchini, sliced

1 red onion, chopped

2 tablespoons balsamic vinegar

1 teaspoon sucralose (optional for a touch of sweetness)

Instructions:

1. **Prepare the Mackerel:** Preheat the grill to medium-high heat. Rub the mackerel fillets with olive oil, dried thyme, paprika, garlic powder, salt, and pepper. Place lemon slices on top of the fillets for added flavor.

2. **Prepare the Vegetables:** Preheat the oven to 425°F (220°C). In a large bowl, toss the baby potatoes, red bell pepper, zucchini, and red onion with olive oil, salt, pepper, and balsamic vinegar. Add sucralose if desired for a touch of sweetness. Spread the vegetables in a single layer on a baking sheet.

3. **Cook the Vegetables:** Roast the vegetables in the preheated oven for 25-30 minutes, or until tender and golden brown, stirring occasionally.

4. **Grill the Mackerel:** While the vegetables are roasting, place the mackerel fillets on the grill. Grill for 4-5 minutes per side, or until the fish is cooked through and flakes easily with a fork.

5. **Serve:** Divide the roasted vegetables among four plates. Top each plate with a grilled mackerel fillet. Garnish with additional lemon slices if desired.

Nutrients (per serving)

Calories: 400 kcal Carbohydrates: 30g Fiber: 6g

Protein: 30g Fat: 20g Sugar: 7g Sodium: 250mg

Calcium: 80mg

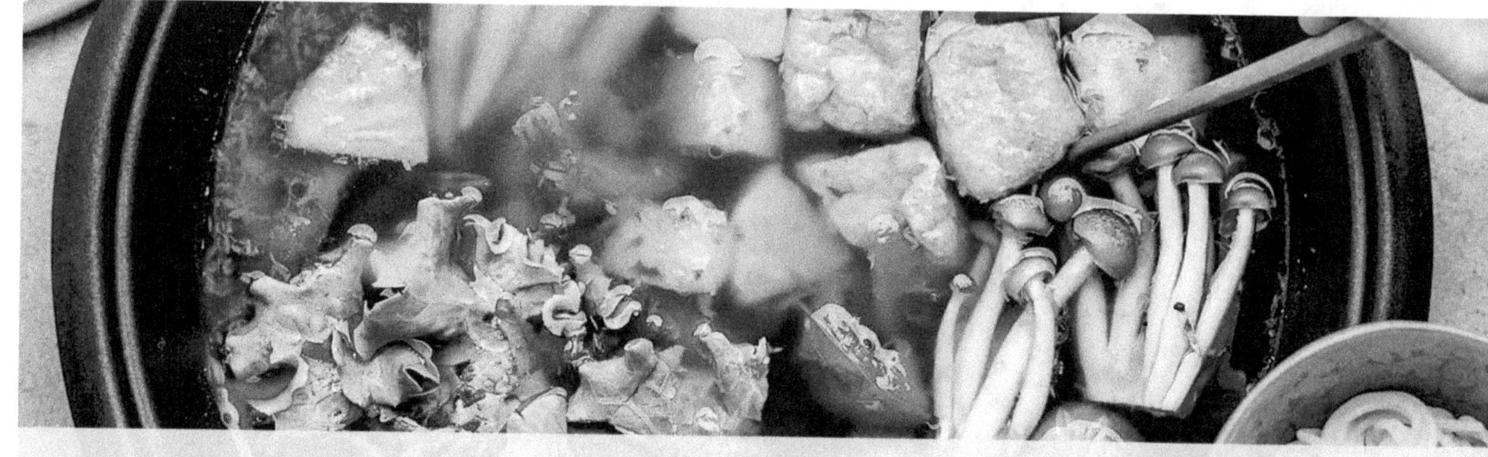

VEGETARIAN HOT POT WITH TOFU AND GREENS

Vegetarian Hot Pot with Tofu and Greens is a flavorful and comforting dish that features a savory broth brimming with fresh vegetables and tender tofu. This recipe is perfect for those looking for a hearty, plant-based meal that's both nutritious and satisfying. Ideal for a cozy dinner with family or friends, it's easy to prepare and offers a warming, nutritious experience.

Serves		Preparation Time		Cooking Time	
4	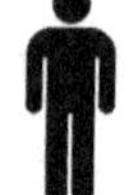	20 minutes		30 minutes	

Ingredients:

1 tablespoon olive oil

1 onion, sliced

3 cloves garlic, minced

1 tablespoon ginger, minced

6 cups vegetable broth

2 tablespoons soy sauce

1 tablespoon rice vinegar

1 teaspoon sucralose (optional for a touch of sweetness)

8 ounces firm tofu, cubed

1 cup shiitake mushrooms, sliced

1 cup baby bok choy, chopped

1 cup snap peas

1 cup carrots, sliced

1 cup broccoli florets

1 cup baby corn

2 green onions, chopped

Fresh cilantro for garnish (optional)

Instructions:

1. **Prepare the Broth:** In a large pot, heat the olive oil over medium heat.Add the sliced onion and cook until softened, about 5 minutes.Stir in the minced garlic and ginger, cooking for an additional 1-2 minutes until fragrant.

2. **Make the Soup Base:** Pour in the vegetable broth, soy sauce, and rice vinegar. Stir well to combine.If using sucralose, add it to the broth for a subtle sweetness. Adjust seasoning with salt and pepper if needed.Bring the broth to a simmer and cook for 10 minutes to allow the flavors to meld.

3. **Add the Tofu and Vegetables:** Gently add the cubed tofu, shiitake mushrooms, baby bok choy, snap peas, carrots, broccoli, and baby corn to the simmering broth.Cook for 10-15 minutes, or until the vegetables are tender and the tofu is heated through.

4. **Serve:** Ladle the hot pot into bowls, garnishing with chopped green onions and fresh cilantro if desired.

Nutrients (per serving)

Calories: 220 kcal Carbohydrates: 30g Fiber: 6g

Protein: 15g Fat: 8g Sugar: 6g Sodium: 600mg

Calcium: 200mg

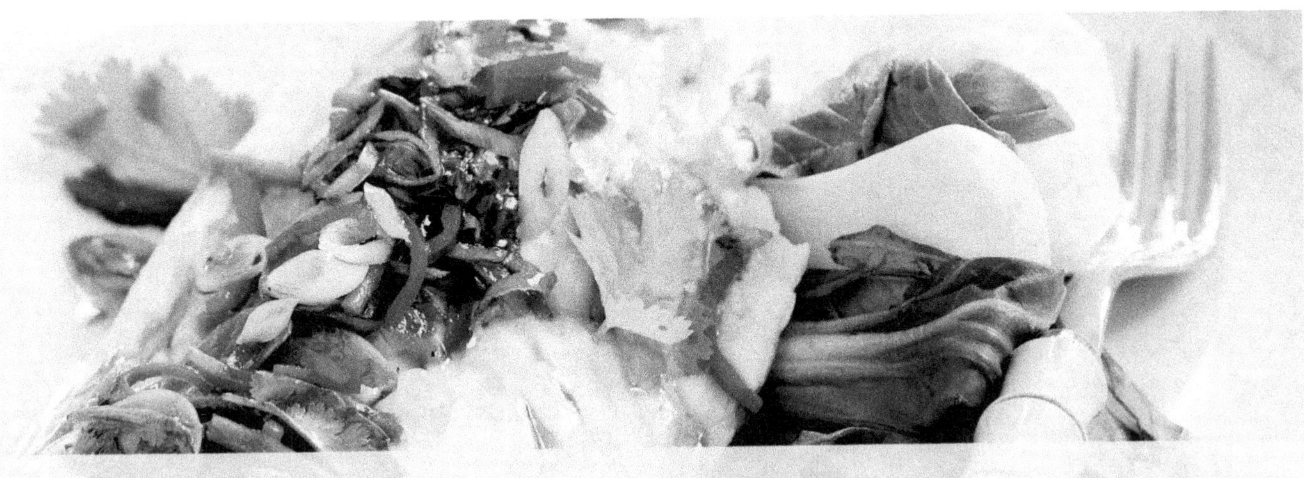

GINGER STEAMED FISH

Ginger Steamed Fish is a light, flavorful dish that highlights the natural taste of the fish while infusing it with the aromatic essence of fresh ginger. Steaming is a healthy cooking method that preserves the nutrients and delicate texture of the fish, making it a perfect choice for a wholesome, satisfying meal. This dish is ideal for those looking for a simple yet elegant option that's rich in flavor and easy to prepare.

Serves	Preparation Time	Cooking Time
4	10 minutes	20 minutes

Ingredients:

4 fish fillets (such as cod, tilapia, or snapper)

2 tablespoons soy sauce

1 tablespoon rice wine or white wine

1 tablespoon sucralose (optional for a hint of sweetness)

2 tablespoons fresh ginger, thinly sliced

2 cloves garlic, minced

2 green onions, sliced

1 tablespoon sesame oil

Fresh cilantro for garnish (optional)

Lemon slices for garnish (optional)

Instructions:

1. **Prepare the Marinade:** In a small bowl, mix the soy sauce, rice wine, and sucralose (if using). Stir well until the sucralose is fully dissolved.
2. **Prepare the Fish:** Pat the fish fillets dry with paper towels. Place them on a heatproof plate that fits inside your steamer. Rub the fillets with the minced garlic and place the thinly sliced ginger on top of each fillet.
3. **Marinate the Fish:** Drizzle the marinade mixture over the fish fillets. Allow to marinate for about 10 minutes.
4. **Steam the Fish:** Set up your steamer and bring the water to a boil. Carefully place the plate with the fish fillets into the steamer basket. Cover and steam the fish for about 15-20 minutes, or until the fish flakes easily with a fork.
5. **Prepare the Garnish:** While the fish is steaming, heat the sesame oil in a small pan over medium heat. Add the sliced green onions and cook for about 1 minute, until fragrant.
6. **Serve:** Once the fish is cooked, remove it from the steamer and carefully transfer to serving plates. Spoon the sautéed green onions and sesame oil over the fish. Garnish with fresh cilantro and lemon slices if desired.

Nutrients (per serving)

Calories: 180 kcal Carbohydrates: 4g Fiber: 1g

Protein: 30g Fat: 4g Sugar: 2g Sodium: 650mg

Calcium: 50mg

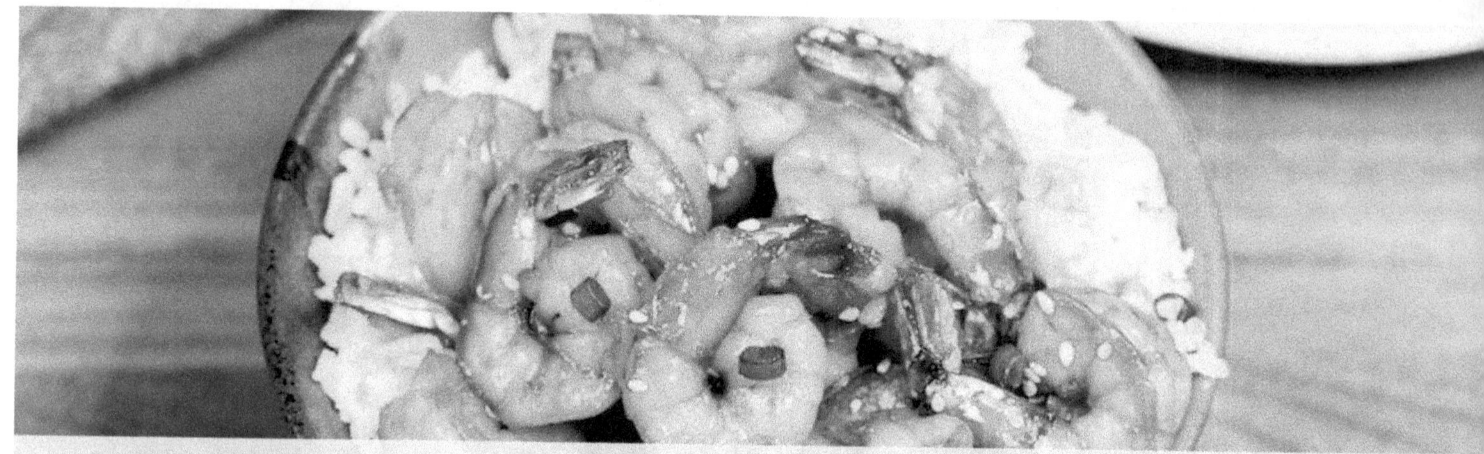

GARLIC SHRIMP WITH BROWN RICE

Garlic Shrimp with Brown Rice is a savory, nutritious dish that combines tender shrimp with the rich flavors of garlic and the wholesome goodness of brown rice. This meal is both satisfying and healthful, offering a balance of protein, fiber, and essential nutrients. Perfect for a quick weeknight dinner or a meal prep option, it's easy to make and packed with flavor.

Serves	**Preparation Time**	**Cooking Time**
4	10 minutes	20 minutes

Ingredients:

1 lb (450g) large shrimp, peeled and deveined
2 tablespoons olive oil
4 cloves garlic, minced
1 teaspoon paprika
1/2 teaspoon crushed red pepper flakes (optional for heat)
1 tablespoon soy sauce
1 tablespoon lemon juice
2 cups cooked brown rice
1/4 cup fresh parsley, chopped (for garnish)
Lemon wedges (for serving)

Instructions:

1. **Prepare the Shrimp:** In a bowl, toss the shrimp with paprika and crushed red pepper flakes (if using).
2. **Cook the Shrimp:** Heat olive oil in a large skillet over medium heat. Add the minced garlic and sauté for about 1 minute, until fragrant but not burnt.Add the seasoned shrimp to the skillet. Cook for about 2-3 minutes on each side, or until the shrimp are pink and opaque.
3. **Add Flavors:** Stir in the soy sauce and lemon juice, cooking for an additional minute to combine the flavors.
4. **Serve:** Divide the cooked brown rice among four plates. Top with the garlic shrimp.Garnish with chopped parsley and serve with lemon wedges on the side.

Nutrients (per serving)

Calories: 350 kcal Carbohydrates: 40g Fiber: 4g
Protein: 30g Fat: 10g Sugar: 2g Sodium: 600mg
Calcium: 60mg

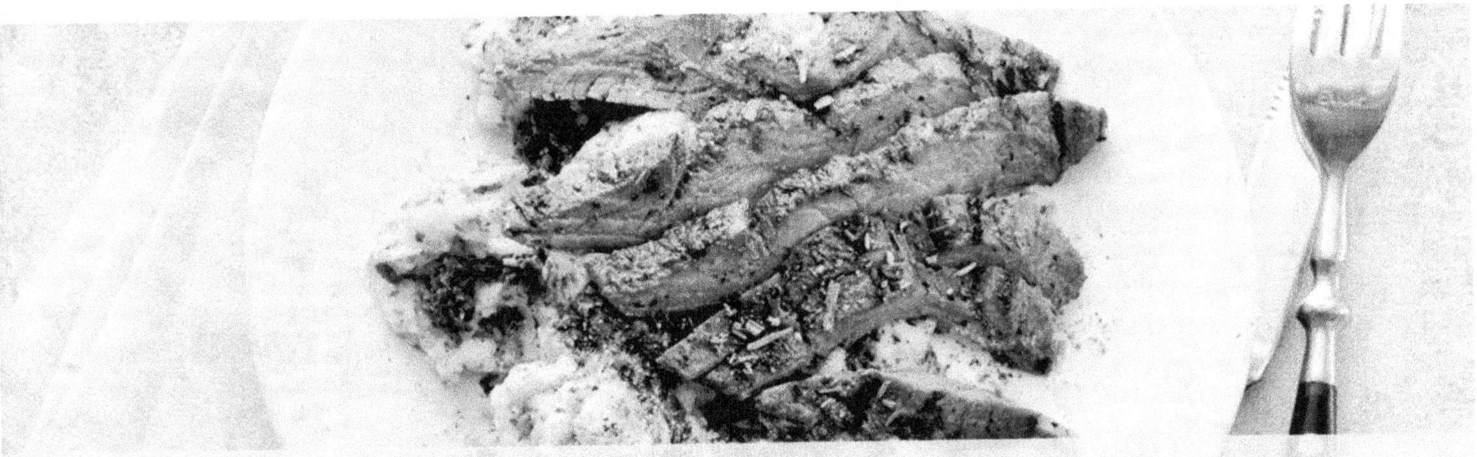

PEPPER GRILLED STEAK WITH MASHED POTATOES

Pepper Grilled Steak with Mashed Potatoes is a classic dish that brings together the savory richness of perfectly grilled steak with creamy, buttery mashed potatoes. The bold peppery flavor of the steak complements the smooth, comforting texture of the mashed potatoes, making this meal a satisfying choice for a hearty dinner. It's a straightforward recipe that delivers both flavor and comfort.

Serves		**Preparation Time**		**Cooking Time**	
4	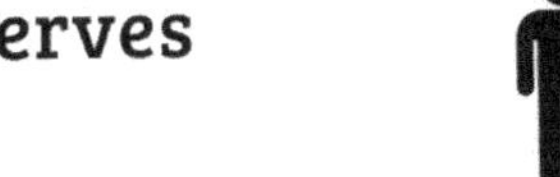	15 minutes		30 minutes	

Ingredients:

For the Steak:

4 (6 oz each) beef sirloin steaks

2 tablespoons olive oil

2 tablespoons freshly ground black pepper

1 tablespoon salt

1 tablespoon garlic powder

1 tablespoon Worcestershire sauce

For the Mashed Potatoes:

4 large russet potatoes, peeled and cubed

1/2 cup milk (or a dairy-free alternative)

1/4 cup unsalted butter

1/4 cup sour cream (or Greek yogurt)

1/2 teaspoon salt

1/4 teaspoon black pepper

2 tablespoons chopped fresh chives (for garnish)

Instructions:

1. **Prepare the Steaks:** Preheat the grill to medium-high heat.Brush the steaks with olive oil and season generously with black pepper, salt, and garlic powder. Drizzle with Worcestershire sauce.Grill the steaks for 4-5 minutes per side for medium-rare, or longer if desired. Use a meat thermometer to check doneness (130°F for medium-rare).Remove from the grill and let the steaks rest for 5 minutes before slicing.

2. **Prepare the Mashed Potatoes:** Place the cubed potatoes in a large pot and cover with water. Bring to a boil and cook until the potatoes are tender, about 15-20 minutes.Drain the potatoes and return them to the pot.Add the milk, butter, and sour cream to the potatoes. Mash until smooth and creamy. Season with salt and black pepper to taste.Garnish with chopped chives.

3. **Serve:** Divide the mashed potatoes among four plates.Top with sliced grilled steak.Serve immediately.

Nutrients (per serving)

Calories: 620 kcal Carbohydrates: 50g Fiber: 5g

Protein: 40g Fat: 30g Sugar: 4g Sodium: 800mg

Calcium: 80mg

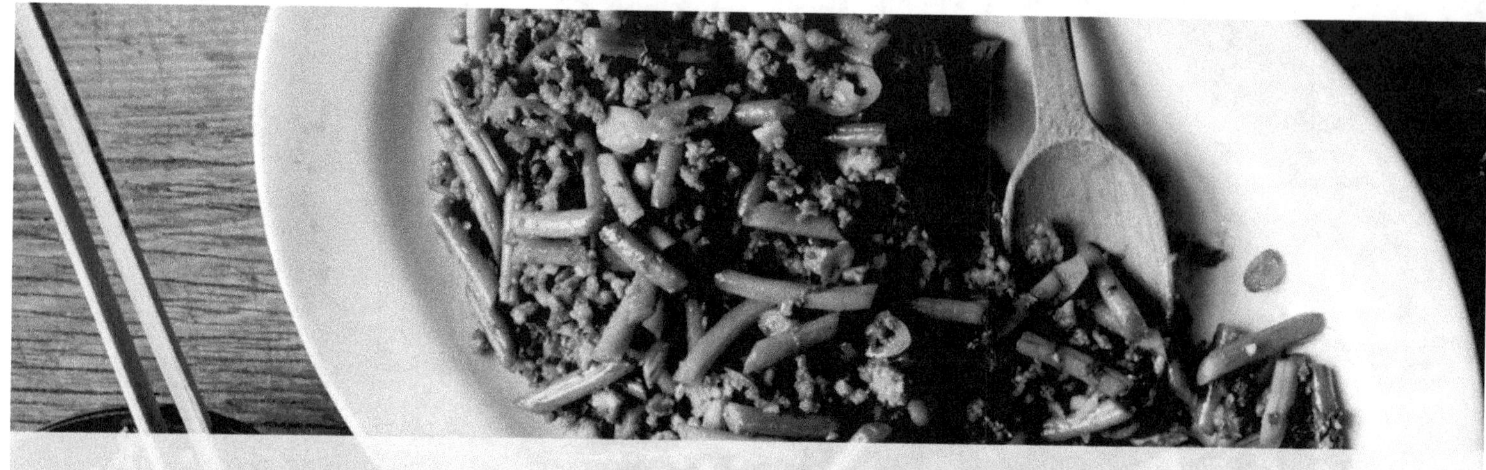

STIR-FRIED PORK WITH GREEN BEANS AND ONIONS

Stir-Fried Pork with Green Beans and Onions is a quick and flavorful dish that brings together tender pork, crisp green beans, and aromatic onions in a savory sauce. This recipe is ideal for a weeknight meal when you need something satisfying and nutritious but don't have a lot of time to cook. The combination of fresh vegetables and seasoned pork creates a delicious, well-balanced meal.

Serves		Preparation Time		Cooking Time	
4		15 minutes		15 minutes	

Ingredients:

1 lb (450g) pork tenderloin, thinly sliced
2 tablespoons vegetable oil
2 cups fresh green beans, trimmed
1 large onion, thinly sliced
3 cloves garlic, minced
1 tablespoon fresh ginger, minced
3 tablespoons soy sauce
2 tablespoons hoisin sauce
1 tablespoon rice vinegar
1 tablespoon sucralose (or to taste)
1/2 cup water
1 teaspoon cornstarch (optional, for thickening)
2 tablespoons chopped fresh cilantro (for garnish)

Instructions:

1. **Prepare the Sauce:** In a small bowl, mix together the soy sauce, hoisin sauce, rice vinegar, and sucralose. Stir until the sucralose is fully dissolved. Set aside.
2. **Cook the Pork:** Heat 1 tablespoon of vegetable oil in a large skillet or wok over medium-high heat.Add the sliced pork and stir-fry until it is cooked through and starts to brown, about 4-5 minutes. Remove the pork from the skillet and set aside.
3. **Cook the Vegetables:** In the same skillet, add the remaining 1 tablespoon of vegetable oil.Add the onions and cook for 2 minutes until they start to soften.Add the garlic and ginger, cooking for an additional 1 minute until fragrant.Add the green beans and stir-fry for about 5 minutes, or until they are tender-crisp.
4. **Combine and Finish:** Return the cooked pork to the skillet with the vegetables.Pour the prepared sauce over the pork and vegetables. Stir to coat everything evenly.If desired, mix the cornstarch with 2 tablespoons of water and add to the skillet to thicken the sauce. Cook for another 1-2 minutes until the sauce has thickened and everything is heated through.
5. **Serve:** Garnish with chopped cilantro.Serve hot over steamed rice or noodles.

Nutrients (per serving)

Calories: 290 kcal Carbohydrates: 20g Fiber: 4g

Protein: 28g Fat: 13g Sugar: 6g Sodium: 750mg

Calcium: 60mg

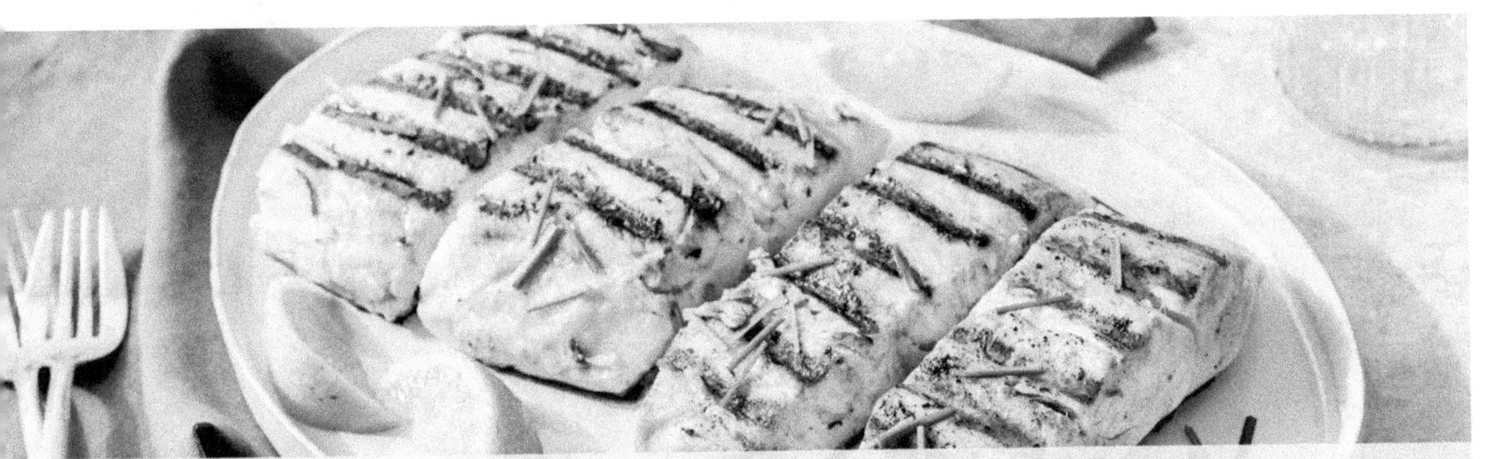

GRILLED SEA BASS WITH CUCUMBER RELISH

Grilled Sea Bass with Cucumber Relish is a light and refreshing dish perfect for a healthy meal. The sea bass is grilled to perfection, and the cucumber relish adds a crisp, tangy contrast that enhances the flavors of the fish. This recipe is ideal for a summer dinner or any time you want a simple yet elegant meal.

Serves	**Preparation Time**	**Cooking Time**
4	15 minutes	10 minutes

Ingredients:

For the Sea Bass:

4 sea bass fillets (about 6 oz each)
2 tablespoons olive oil
1 teaspoon lemon juice
1 teaspoon dried oregano
Salt and pepper, to taste

For the Cucumber Relish:

1 large cucumber, peeled, seeded, and diced
1/4 cup red onion, finely chopped
1 tablespoon fresh dill, chopped (or 1 teaspoon dried dill)
1 tablespoon lemon juice
1 tablespoon sucralose (or to taste)
Salt and pepper, to taste

Instructions:

1. **Prepare the Sea Bass:** Preheat the grill to medium-high heat. In a small bowl, mix together the olive oil, lemon juice, dried oregano, salt, and pepper.Brush the sea bass fillets with the oil mixture on both sides.Place the fillets on the grill and cook for 4-5 minutes per side, or until the fish flakes easily with a fork and has grill marks.

2. **Prepare the Cucumber Relish:** In a medium bowl, combine the diced cucumber, red onion, dill, lemon juice, and sucralose.Season with salt and pepper to taste.Stir well to combine and let it sit for at least 10 minutes to allow the flavors to meld.

3. **Serve:** Remove the sea bass from the grill and place on serving plates.Top each fillet with a generous spoonful of cucumber relish.Garnish with extra dill, if desired.

Nutrients (per serving)

Calories: 220 kcal Carbohydrates: 8g Fiber: 1g

Protein: 24g Fat: 10g Sugar: 5g Sodium: 120mg

Calcium: 40mg

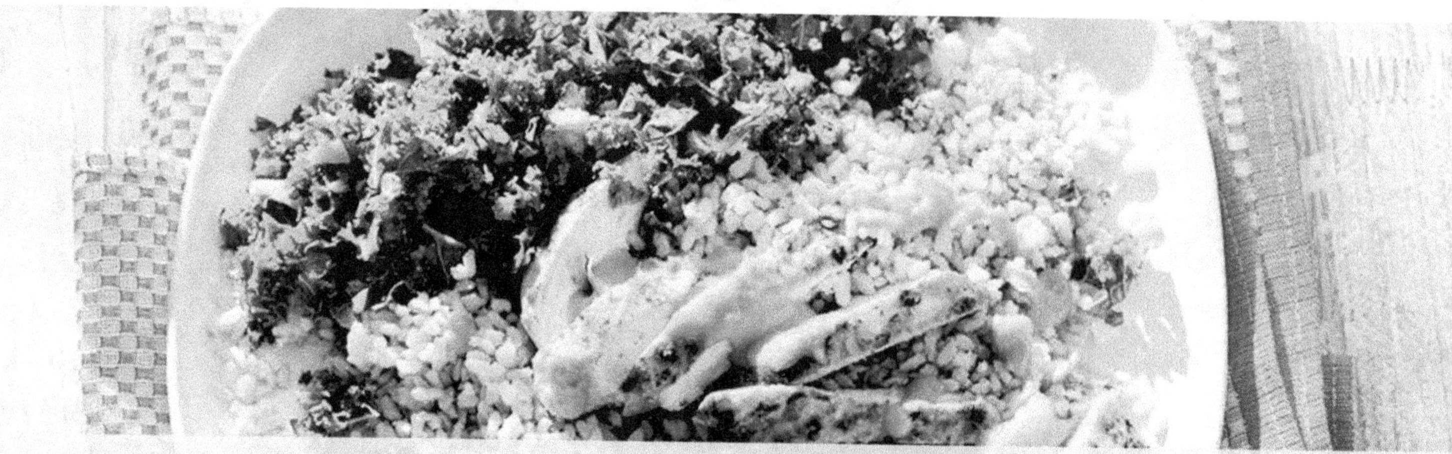

PAN-SEARED CHICKEN WITH KALE AND BROWN RICE

Pan-Seared Chicken with Kale and Brown Rice is a wholesome and satisfying dish that combines tender chicken with nutritious kale and hearty brown rice. This recipe provides a balanced meal with lean protein, fiber, and essential vitamins, making it an ideal choice for a healthy weeknight dinner.

Serves		**Preparation Time**		**Cooking Time**	
4		15 minutes		30 minutes	

Ingredients:

For the Chicken:
4 boneless, skinless chicken breasts (about 6 oz each)
2 tablespoons olive oil
1 teaspoon paprika
1 teaspoon garlic powder
1/2 teaspoon onion powder
Salt and pepper, to taste

For the Kale and Brown Rice:
1 cup brown rice
2 cups water or low-sodium chicken broth
4 cups kale, stems removed and leaves chopped
1 tablespoon olive oil
2 cloves garlic, minced
1/2 teaspoon crushed red pepper flakes (optional)
Salt and pepper, to taste
Juice of 1 lemon

Instructions:

1. **Cook the Brown Rice:** In a medium pot, bring water or chicken broth to a boil. Add the brown rice, reduce heat to low, cover, and simmer for 45 minutes, or until the rice is tender and the liquid is absorbed. Remove from heat and let it sit covered for 5 minutes, then fluff with a fork.
2. **Prepare the Chicken:** While the rice is cooking, season the chicken breasts with paprika, garlic powder, onion powder, salt, and pepper. Heat olive oil in a large skillet over medium-high heat. Add the chicken breasts and cook for 6-7 minutes per side, or until the chicken is golden brown and cooked through (internal temperature should reach 165°F or 74°C). Remove the chicken from the skillet and let it rest for a few minutes before slicing.
3. **Prepare the Kale:** In the same skillet, add 1 tablespoon of olive oil over medium heat.Add the minced garlic and crushed red pepper flakes (if using), and cook for about 1 minute until fragrant.Add the chopped kale to the skillet and sauté for 5-6 minutes, or until wilted and tender.Season with salt and pepper, and squeeze the lemon juice over the kale. Stir to combine.
4. **Serve:** Divide the brown rice among four plates.Top with a portion of sautéed kale and a sliced chicken breast.Garnish with extra lemon wedges if desired.

Nutrients (per serving)

Calories: 400 kcal Carbohydrates: 40g Fiber: 6g
Protein: 32g Fat: 14g Sugar: 3g Sodium: 150mg
Calcium: 120mg

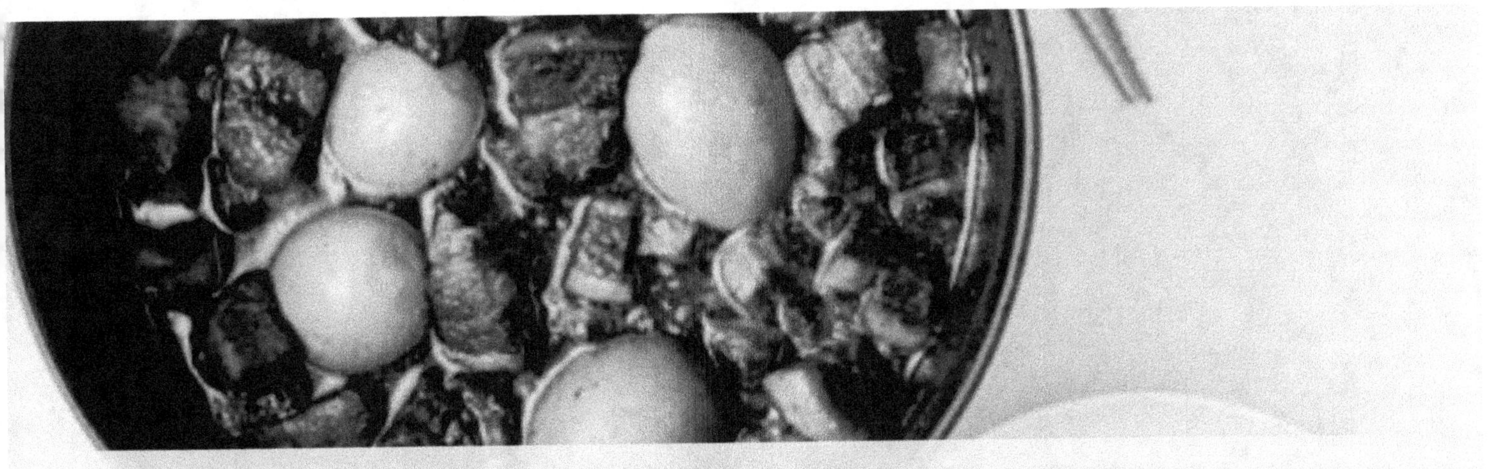

BRAISED PORK WITH EGGS AND WATER SPINACH

Braised Pork with Eggs and Water Spinach is a savory and comforting dish that pairs tender braised pork with rich, flavorful eggs and nutritious water spinach. This dish offers a delightful combination of textures and flavors, providing a balanced and satisfying meal that's perfect for a family dinner or a special occasion.

Serves		Preparation Time		Cooking Time	
4		15 minutes		90 minutes	

Ingredients:

For the Braised Pork:

1.5 lbs (680g) pork belly, cut into 1-inch cubes

2 tablespoons vegetable oil

4 cloves garlic, minced

1 tablespoon ginger, minced

1/4 cup soy sauce

1/4 cup hoisin sauce

1/4 cup rice wine or dry sherry

1 tablespoon brown sugar

2 cups water

2 star anise

1 cinnamon stick

4 hard-boiled eggs, peeled

For the Water Spinach:

4 cups water spinach, chopped (substitute with other leafy greens if unavailable)

2 tablespoons vegetable oil

2 cloves garlic, minced

Salt and pepper, to taste

Instructions:

1. **Braise the Pork:** Heat vegetable oil in a large pot or Dutch oven over medium-high heat.Add the pork belly cubes and sear until browned on all sides, about 5-7 minutes.Remove the pork from the pot and set aside.In the same pot, add minced garlic and ginger, and cook for 1 minute until fragrant.Return the pork to the pot and add soy sauce, hoisin sauce, rice wine (or sherry), brown sugar, and water. Stir to combine.Add star anise and cinnamon stick.Bring to a boil, then reduce heat to low, cover, and simmer for 1 hour, stirring occasionally.After 1 hour, add the hard-boiled eggs to the pot, cover, and continue simmering for an additional 30 minutes. The pork should be tender and the sauce thickened.

2. **Prepare the Water Spinach:** Heat vegetable oil in a large skillet over medium heat.Add minced garlic and cook for about 1 minute until fragrant.Add the chopped water spinach and sauté for 3-4 minutes, or until wilted and tender.Season with salt and pepper to taste.

3. **Serve:** Divide the braised pork, eggs, and sauce among four plates.Serve with a side of sautéed water spinach.

Nutrients (per serving)

Calories: 550 kcal Carbohydrates: 20g Fiber: 3g

Protein: 35g Fat: 35g Sugar: 8g Sodium: 900mg

Calcium: 120mg

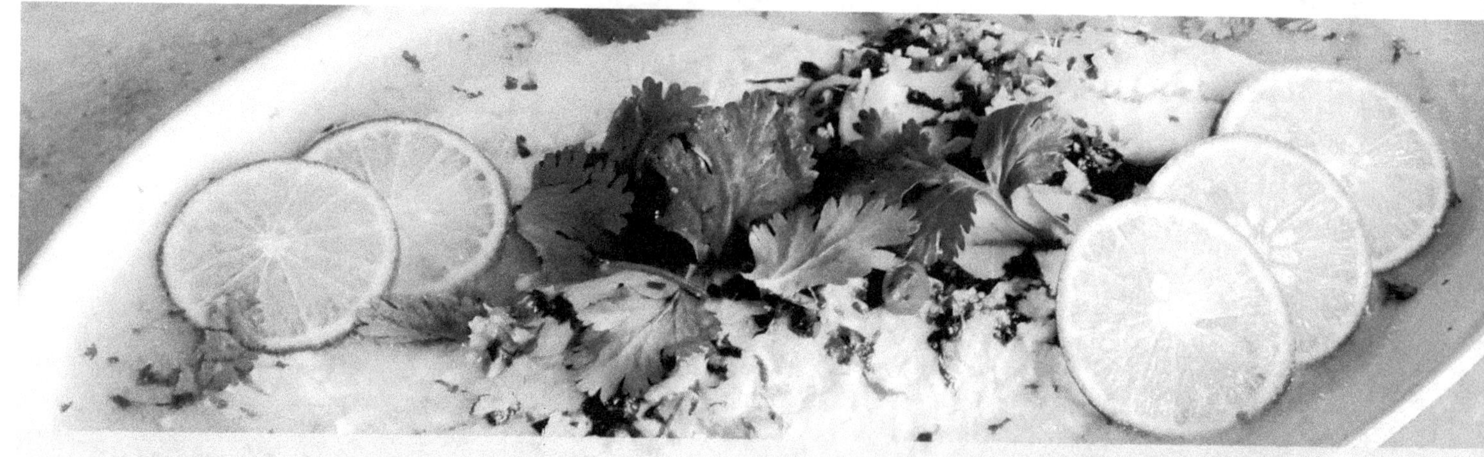

STEAMED FISH WITH LEMONGRASS AND FISH SAUCE

Steamed Fish with Lemongrass and Fish Sauce is a light yet flavorful dish that highlights the delicate taste of fish enhanced with aromatic lemongrass and savory fish sauce. This dish is perfect for a healthy meal, offering a balance of fresh flavors and simple preparation. It's an excellent choice for those who enjoy light, aromatic, and health-conscious recipes.

Serves	Preparation Time	Cooking Time
4	15 minutes	20 minutes

Ingredients:

4 fish fillets (such as cod, tilapia, or snapper), about 6 oz (170g) each

2 stalks lemongrass, trimmed and sliced thinly

4 cloves garlic, minced

2 tablespoons fish sauce

1 tablespoon soy sauce

1 tablespoon rice wine or dry sherry

1 teaspoon sugar (optional)

1 small red chili, thinly sliced (optional, for a bit of heat)

2 tablespoons fresh cilantro, chopped (for garnish)

1 tablespoon vegetable oil

1 lime, cut into wedges (for serving)

Instructions:

1. **Prepare the Fish:** Rinse the fish fillets under cold water and pat them dry with paper towels.Season the fillets lightly with salt and pepper.
2. **Prepare the Steaming Setup:** Fill a large pot or steamer with about 1-2 inches of water and bring it to a boil.Place a steaming rack or heatproof plate inside the pot.
3. **Make the Lemongrass Mixture:** In a small bowl, mix together the minced garlic, fish sauce, soy sauce, rice wine (or sherry), and sugar (if using).Add the sliced lemongrass and red chili (if using) to the mixture.
4. **Steam the Fish:** Place the fish fillets on the steaming rack or heatproof plate.Pour the lemongrass mixture over the fish fillets.Drizzle with vegetable oil.Cover the pot with a lid and steam the fish for about 15-20 minutes, or until the fish flakes easily with a fork.
5. **Garnish and Serve:** Carefully remove the fish from the pot.Garnish with fresh cilantro.Serve with lime wedges on the side.

Nutrients (per serving)

Calories: 220 kcal Carbohydrates: 6g Fiber: 1g

Protein: 25g Fat: 10g Sugar: 2g Sodium: 800mg

Calcium: 50mg

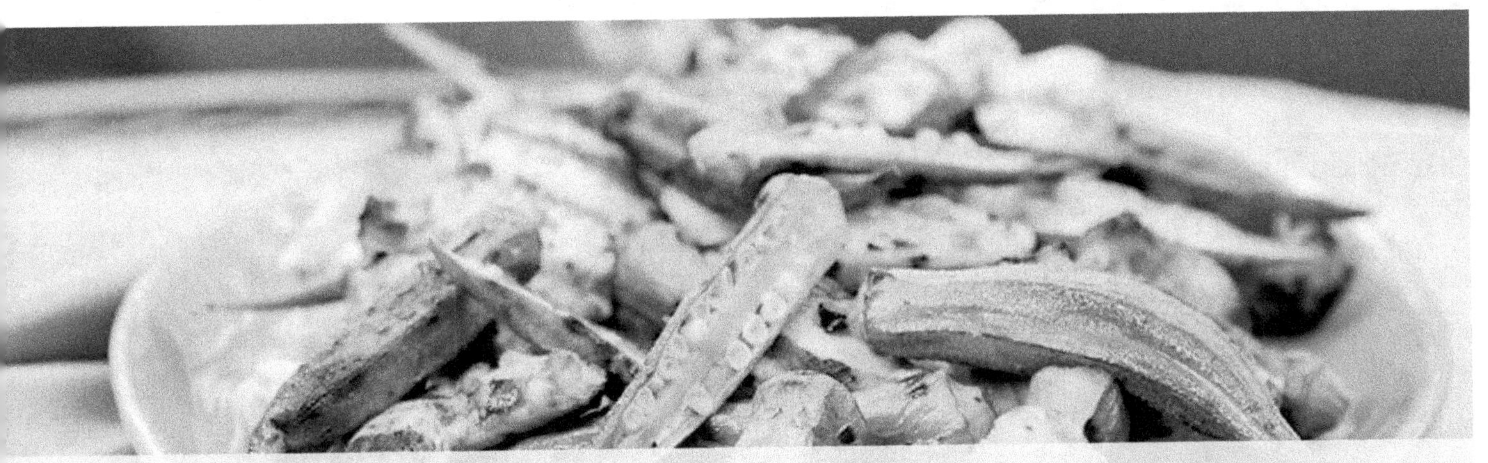

GRILLED LEMONGRASS CHICKEN WITH OKRA

Grilled Lemongrass Chicken with Okra is a savory and aromatic dish that combines tender chicken marinated in lemongrass, garlic, and spices with perfectly grilled okra. This healthy meal is full of vibrant flavors and provides a nutrient-rich option, making it perfect for meal prep or a light dinner.

Serves	Preparation Time	Cooking Time
4	 20 minutes	 15 minutes

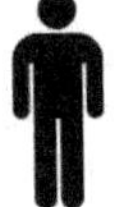

Ingredients:

4 boneless, skinless chicken thighs (about 1 lb / 450g)
2 stalks lemongrass, finely chopped
3 cloves garlic, minced
1 tablespoon fish sauce
1 tablespoon soy sauce
1 tablespoon olive oil (for marinade)
1 tablespoon honey (or sucralose equivalent)
1 teaspoon ground turmeric
1 teaspoon ground black pepper
1 lime (juice for marinating and wedges for serving)
12-16 fresh okra, trimmed
1 tablespoon olive oil (for grilling)
Salt and pepper to taste
Fresh cilantro for garnish

Instructions:

1. **Marinate the Chicken:** In a large bowl, mix together the chopped lemongrass, minced garlic, fish sauce, soy sauce, olive oil, honey (or sucralose), turmeric, black pepper, and lime juice.Add the chicken thighs to the marinade, making sure they are evenly coated. Cover and refrigerate for at least 1 hour (or up to 4 hours for better flavor).
2. **Prepare the Okra:** Toss the trimmed okra with 1 tablespoon of olive oil, salt, and pepper.
3. **Grill the Chicken and Okra:** Preheat the grill to medium-high heat.Grill the marinated chicken thighs for about 5-7 minutes on each side, or until fully cooked through and the internal temperature reaches 165°F (75°C).Grill the okra alongside the chicken, turning occasionally, for about 8-10 minutes or until they are tender and slightly charred.
4. **Serve:** Remove the chicken and okra from the grill and let the chicken rest for 5 minutes before slicing.Garnish with fresh cilantro and serve with lime wedges on the side.

Nutrients (per serving)

Calories: 320 kcal Carbohydrates: 8g Fiber: 3g

Protein: 28g Fat: 18g Sugar: 4g Sodium: 680mg

Calcium: 50mg

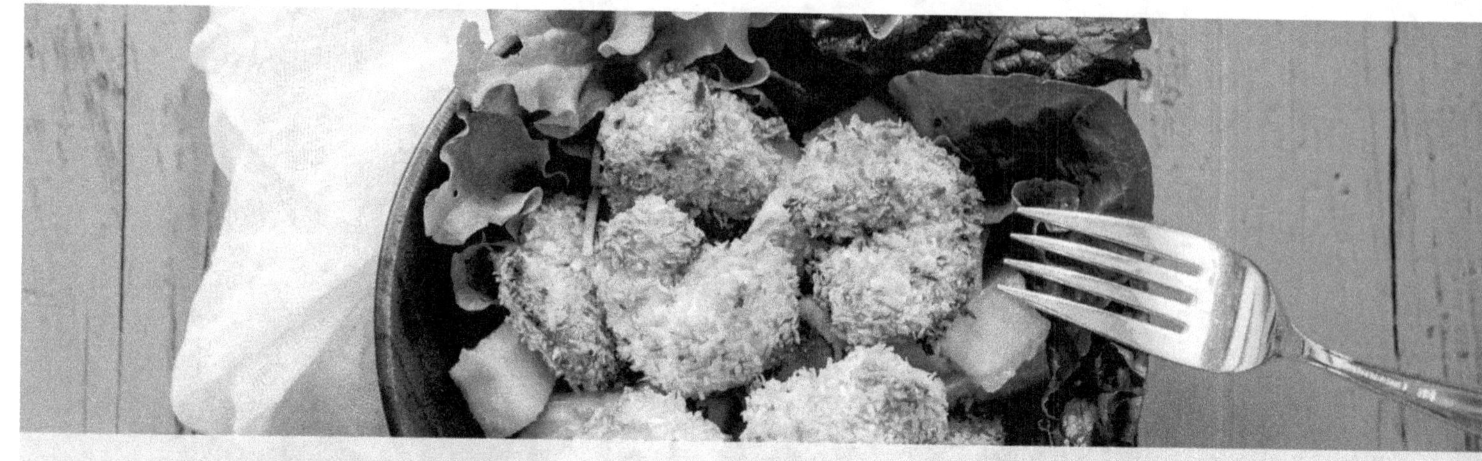

CRISPY FRIED SHRIMP WITH MANGO SALAD

Crispy Fried Shrimp with Mango Salad is a delightful combination of crunchy, golden-fried shrimp and a refreshing, zesty mango salad. The sweetness of ripe mangoes, combined with the crispiness of the shrimp, creates a balanced, tropical-inspired dish perfect for a healthy lunch or light dinner.

Serves		Preparation Time	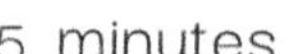	Cooking Time	
4		20 minutes		15 minutes	

Ingredients:

For the Shrimp:

1 lb (450g) large shrimp, peeled and deveined

1/2 cup almond flour (or whole-wheat flour)

1/2 cup breadcrumbs (use gluten-free if needed)

1 large egg, beaten

1 teaspoon garlic powder

1 teaspoon paprika

Salt and pepper to taste

Olive oil (for frying)

For the Mango Salad:

2 ripe mangoes, peeled and diced

1 cucumber, thinly sliced

1/2 red onion, thinly sliced

1 red bell pepper, diced

1/4 cup fresh cilantro, chopped

Juice of 1 lime

1 tablespoon olive oil

1 teaspoon honey (or sucralose equivalent)

Salt and pepper to taste

Instructions:

1. **Prepare the Shrimp:** In one bowl, mix the almond flour, breadcrumbs, garlic powder, paprika, salt, and pepper. In another bowl, beat the egg. Dip each shrimp into the beaten egg, then coat it with the flour-breadcrumb mixture, pressing gently to ensure an even coating.
2. **Fry the Shrimp:** Heat a large skillet over medium heat and add enough olive oil to cover the bottom of the pan. Fry the shrimp in batches, about 2-3 minutes per side, until golden brown and crispy.
3. Remove and drain on a paper towel-lined plate.
4. **Make the Mango Salad:** In a large bowl, combine the diced mangoes, cucumber, red onion, bell pepper, and cilantro. In a small bowl, whisk together the lime juice, olive oil, honey (or sucralose), salt, and pepper. Pour the dressing over the mango salad and toss to combine.
5. **Serve:** Plate the crispy shrimp alongside the mango salad or serve them on top of the salad for a complete meal. Garnish with extra cilantro and lime wedges if desired.

Nutrients (per serving)

Calories: 380 kcal Carbohydrates: 25g Fiber: 4g

Protein: 24g Fat: 18g Sugar: 14g Sodium: 480mg

Calcium: 90mg

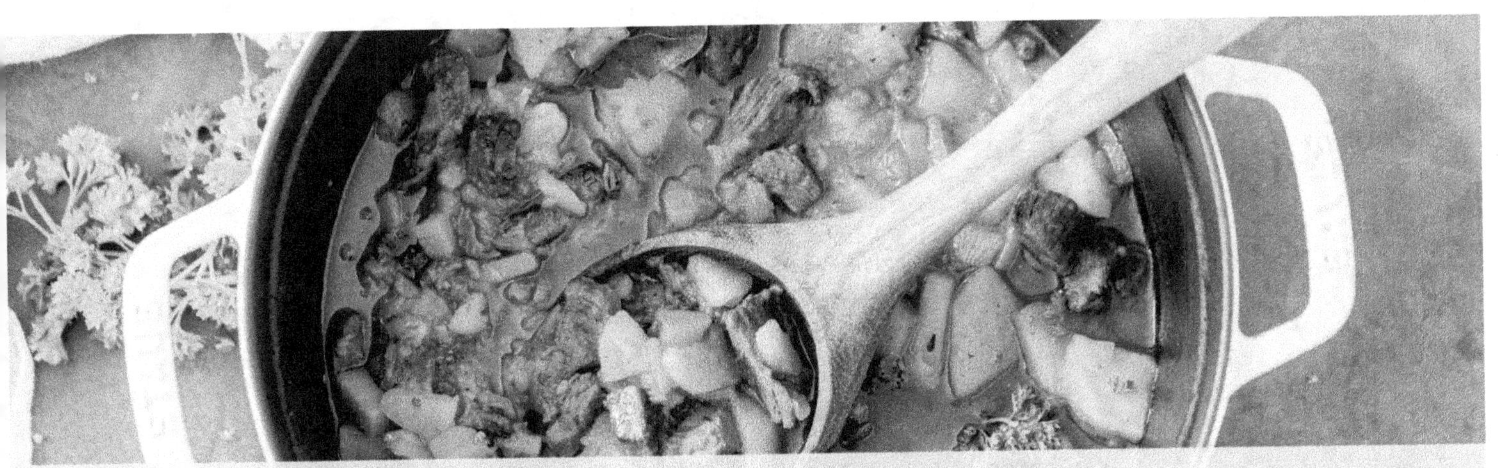

BRAISED BEEF WITH POTATOES

Braised Beef with Potatoes is a hearty and comforting dish, perfect for a satisfying family dinner. Tender beef slowly braised in a rich, flavorful broth with soft, melt-in-your-mouth potatoes creates a classic meal that's both nutritious and delicious. Ideal for meal prepping or batch cooking, this dish only gets better with time as the flavors develop.

Serves		**Preparation Time**		**Cooking Time**	
4		20 minutes		2 hours	

Ingredients:

- 1.5 lbs (680g) beef chuck, cut into large chunks
- 4 large potatoes, peeled and quartered
- 2 carrots, chopped
- 1 large onion, diced
- 3 garlic cloves, minced
- 2 cups beef broth (low-sodium)
- 1 cup water
- 2 tablespoons tomato paste
- 2 tablespoons olive oil
- 1 tablespoon soy sauce (low-sodium)
- 1 teaspoon dried thyme
- 2 bay leaves
- Salt and pepper to taste
- Fresh parsley, chopped (for garnish)

Instructions:

1. **Prepare the Beef:** Season the beef chunks with salt and pepper. Heat olive oil in a large pot over medium-high heat. Sear the beef on all sides until browned, about 5-6 minutes. Remove and set aside.
2. **Sauté Vegetables:** In the same pot, add the diced onions, minced garlic, and carrots. Sauté for 3-4 minutes until softened.
3. **Build the Broth:** Stir in the tomato paste and cook for another 1-2 minutes. Add the beef broth, water, soy sauce, thyme, and bay leaves. Stir to combine.
4. **Braise the Beef:** Return the seared beef to the pot. Bring the liquid to a boil, then reduce heat to low. Cover the pot and let the beef simmer for 1.5 hours.
5. **Add Potatoes:** After 1.5 hours, add the quartered potatoes to the pot. Stir to ensure they are submerged in the broth. Continue to simmer for another 30 minutes, or until the beef is tender and the potatoes are cooked through.
6. **Serve:** Remove the bay leaves and adjust the seasoning with salt and pepper if needed. Serve the braised beef and potatoes in bowls, garnished with fresh parsley.

Nutrients (per serving)

Calories: 480 kcal Carbohydrates: 35g Fiber: 6g

Protein: 32g Fat: 22g Sugar: 4g Sodium: 540mg

Calcium: 60mg

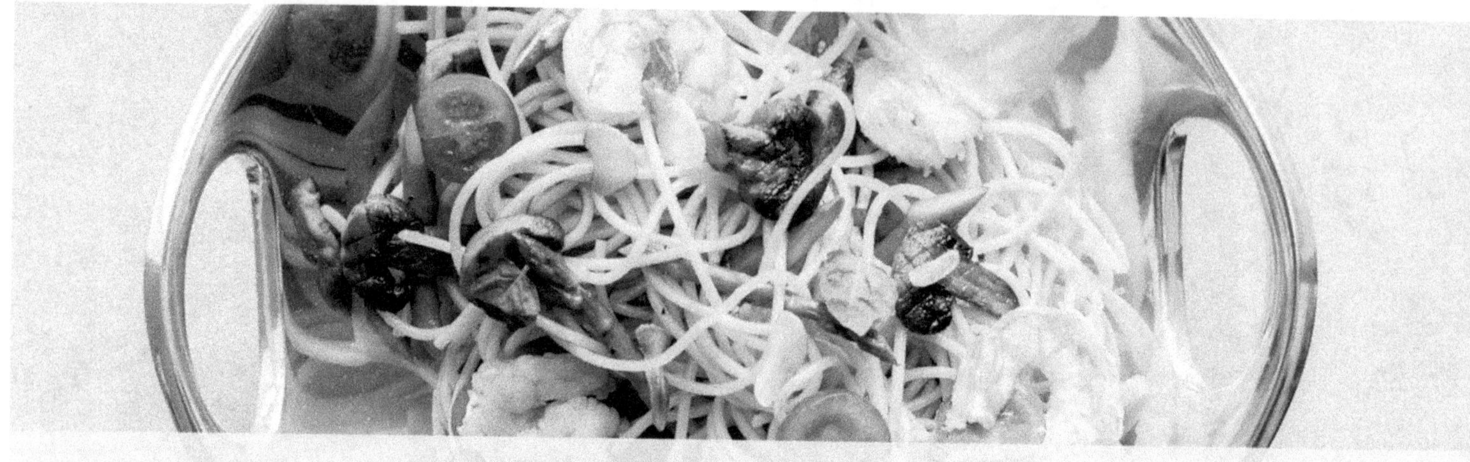

BROWN RICE PASTA WITH SHRIMP AND VEGETABLES

Brown Rice Pasta with Shrimp and Vegetables is a wholesome, gluten-free meal that's both satisfying and nutritious. Packed with lean protein from shrimp, fiber-rich vegetables, and healthy carbs from brown rice pasta, this dish is perfect for

Serves

4

Preparation Time

15 minutes

Cooking Time

20 minutes

Ingredients:

8 oz (225g) brown rice pasta

1 lb (450g) shrimp, peeled and deveined

1 bell pepper, sliced

1 zucchini, sliced

1 cup broccoli florets

2 garlic cloves, minced

2 tablespoons olive oil

1 tablespoon lemon juice

1 teaspoon dried oregano

1 teaspoon paprika

Salt and pepper to taste

Fresh parsley, chopped (for garnish)

Instructions:

1. **Cook the Pasta:** Bring a large pot of salted water to a boil. Add the brown rice pasta and cook according to package instructions until al dente (usually about 8-10 minutes). Drain and set aside.
2. **Prepare the Shrimp:** In a medium bowl, toss the shrimp with paprika, oregano, salt, and pepper. Set aside.
3. **Sauté Vegetables:** Heat 1 tablespoon of olive oil in a large skillet over medium heat. Add the garlic and sauté for 1 minute until fragrant.Add the bell pepper, zucchini, and broccoli florets. Sauté for 5-6 minutes until the vegetables are tender but still crisp.
4. **Cook the Shrimp:** In the same skillet, push the vegetables to the side and add the remaining 1 tablespoon of olive oil.Add the shrimp and cook for 2-3 minutes on each side, or until the shrimp turn pink and are fully cooked.
5. **Combine Everything:** Stir the cooked pasta into the skillet with the shrimp and vegetables. Drizzle with lemon juice and toss to combine.Adjust seasoning with salt and pepper if needed.
6. **Serve:** Divide the pasta between bowls and garnish with fresh parsley. Serve warm.

Nutrients (per serving)

Calories: 350 kcal Carbohydrates: 40g Fiber: 6g

Protein: 28g Fat: 10g Sugar: 3g Sodium: 560mg

Calcium: 120mg

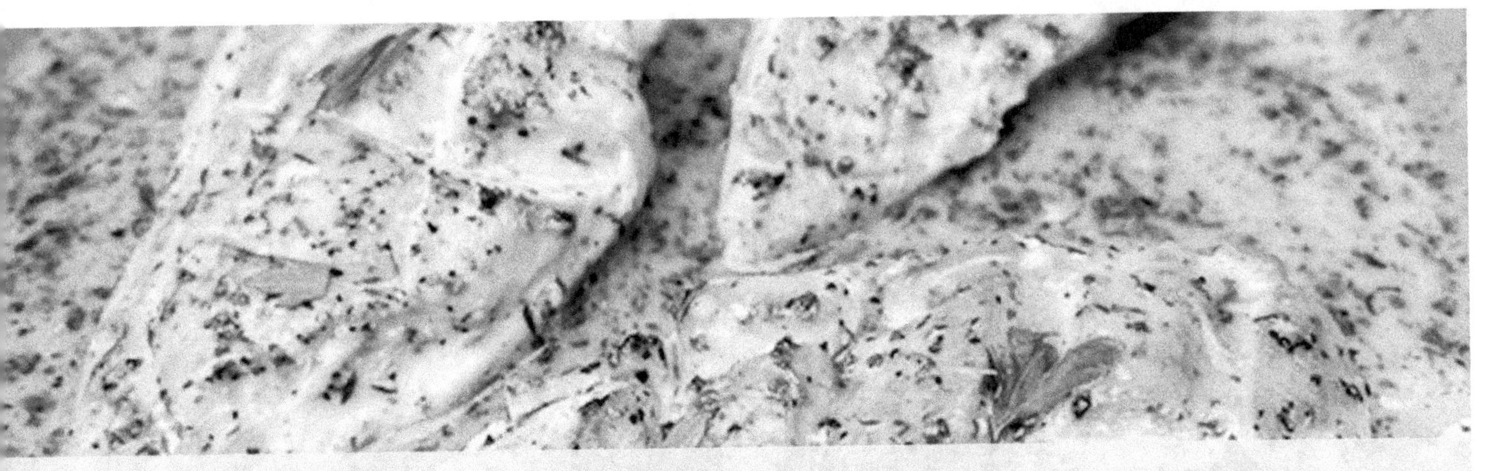

PAN-SEARED CHICKEN WITH LEMON SAUCE

Pan-Seared Chicken with Lemon Sauce is a simple yet flavorful dish, perfect for a healthy weeknight dinner or meal prep. The chicken is juicy with a golden crust, complemented by a tangy lemon sauce that adds brightness without overpowering the meal. Pair it with steamed veggies or brown rice for a well-rounded, nutritious dish.

Serves		Preparation Time		Cooking Time	
4	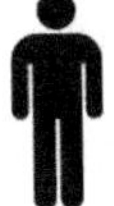	10 minutes		20 minutes	

Ingredients:

4 boneless, skinless chicken breasts

2 tablespoons olive oil

1 tablespoon butter

1 garlic clove, minced

1/2 cup low-sodium chicken broth

1/4 cup lemon juice (freshly squeezed)

1 teaspoon lemon zest

1 teaspoon dried thyme

Salt and pepper, to taste

Fresh parsley, chopped (for garnish)

Instructions:

1. **Season the Chicken:** Pat the chicken breasts dry with paper towels. Season both sides with salt, pepper, and thyme.
2. **Pan-Sear the Chicken:** Heat olive oil in a large skillet over medium-high heat. Once hot, add the chicken breasts to the skillet.Cook for 6-7 minutes on each side, or until golden brown and cooked through (internal temperature should reach 165°F / 75°C). Remove the chicken from the skillet and set aside.
3. **Make the Lemon Sauce:** In the same skillet, reduce the heat to medium and add butter. Once melted, add the minced garlic and sauté for 1 minute until fragrant.Pour in the chicken broth, lemon juice, and lemon zest, stirring to combine. Simmer the sauce for 2-3 minutes to reduce slightly.
4. **Combine:** Return the chicken breasts to the skillet, spooning the sauce over the top. Let them simmer in the lemon sauce for another 2-3 minutes to absorb the flavors.
5. **Serve:** Plate the chicken and spoon additional lemon sauce over each piece. Garnish with fresh parsley and serve alongside your choice of sides.

Nutrients (per serving)

Calories: 280 kcal Carbohydrates: 2g Fiber: 0g

Protein: 34g Fat: 14g Sugar: 0g Sodium: 320mg

Calcium: 30mg

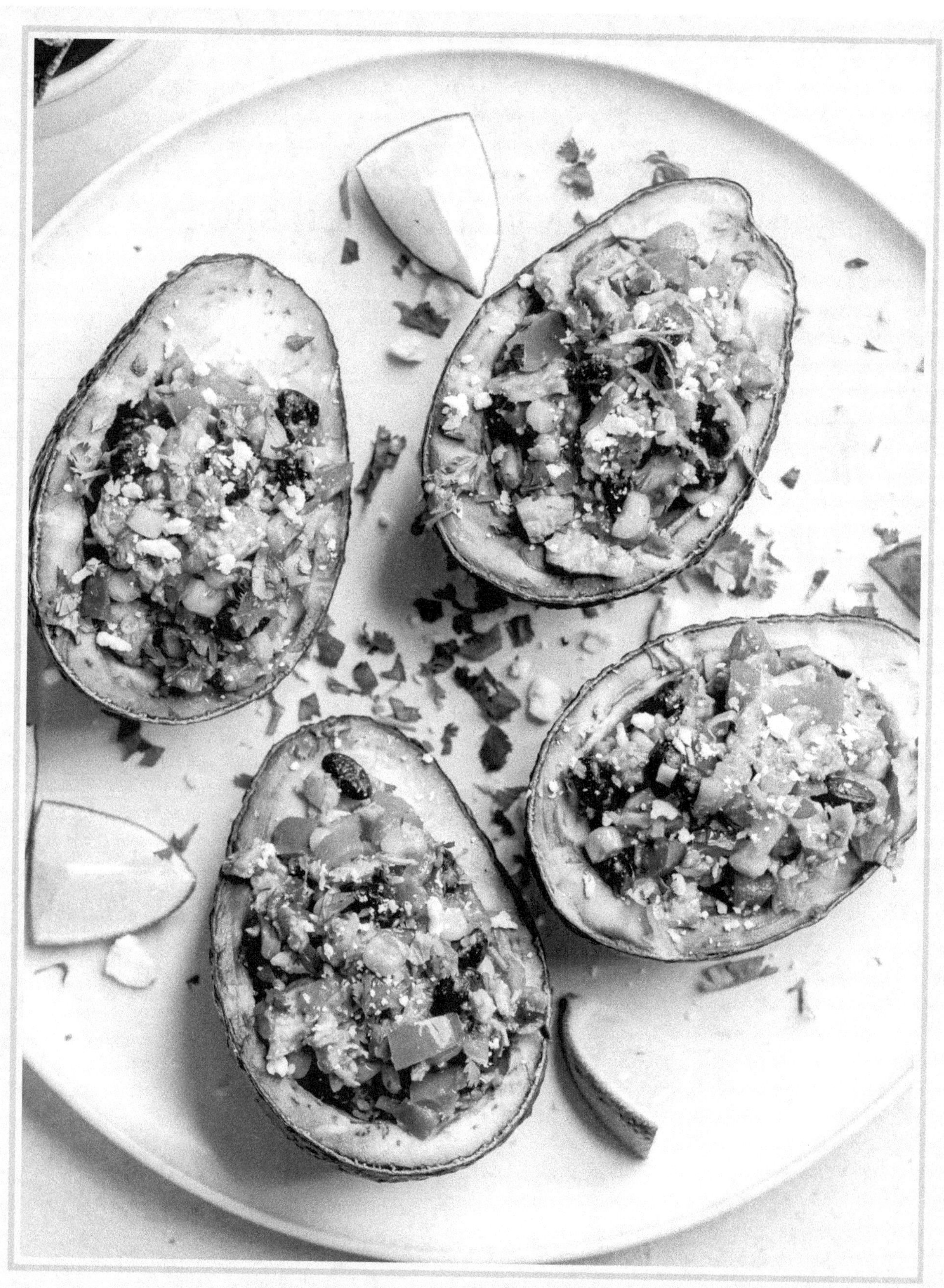

TABLE OF CONTENTS

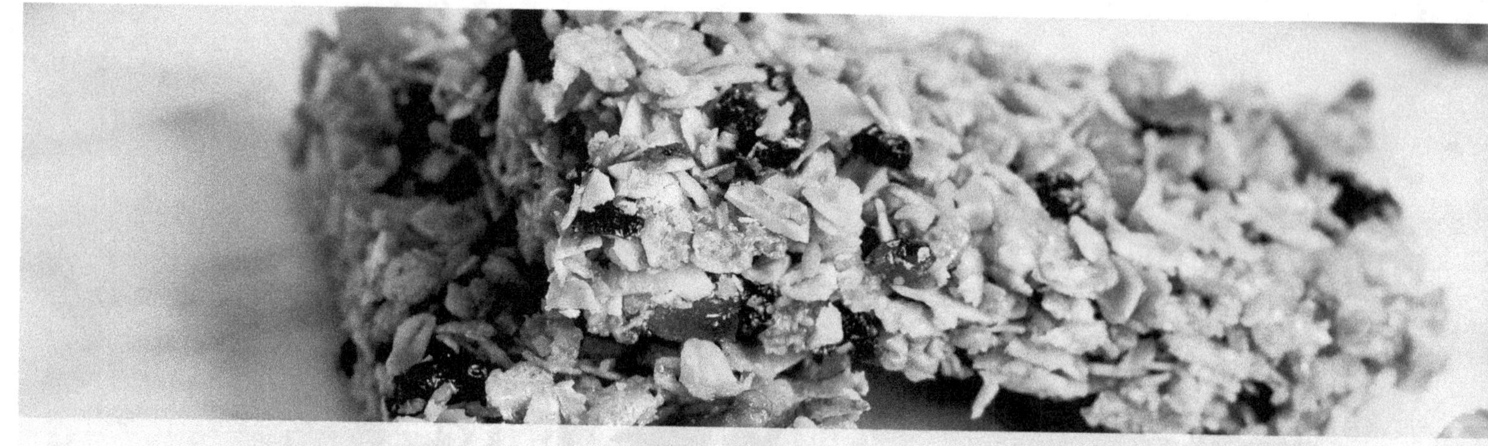

HOMEMADE GRANOLA BARS WITH HONEY

Homemade Granola Bars with Honey are a perfect grab-and-go snack packed with wholesome ingredients. These bars are naturally sweetened with honey, making them a healthy alternative to store-bought versions. They are chewy, flavorful, and can be customized with your favorite nuts, seeds, and dried fruits.

Serves	Preparation Time	Cooking Time
12	10 minutes	25 minute

Ingredients:

2 cups rolled oats
1/2 cup almonds, chopped
1/4 cup sunflower seeds
1/4 cup dried cranberries
1/4 cup honey
1/4 cup peanut butter (or almond butter)
1 teaspoon vanilla extract
1/4 teaspoon salt
1 tablespoon chia seeds (optional)
1/4 cup dark chocolate chips (optional)

Instructions:

1. **Preheat the Oven:** Preheat your oven to 325°F (165°C) and line an 8x8-inch baking pan with parchment paper.
2. **Mix the Dry Ingredients:** In a large bowl, combine the rolled oats, chopped almonds, sunflower seeds, dried cranberries, and chia seeds (if using).
3. **Prepare the Wet Mixture:** In a small saucepan, gently heat the honey and peanut butter over low heat, stirring until smooth and combined. Remove from heat and stir in the vanilla extract and salt.
4. **Combine:** Pour the honey-peanut butter mixture over the dry ingredients. Stir until everything is evenly coated and sticky. If using chocolate chips, fold them in at this stage.
5. **Transfer to Baking Pan:** Press the mixture firmly into the prepared baking pan, ensuring an even layer. Use the back of a spoon or your hands to pack it down tightly.
6. **Bake:** Bake for 20-25 minutes, or until the edges are golden brown. Remove from the oven and allow the bars to cool in the pan for 10 minutes.
7. **Cut and Serve:** Once slightly cooled, lift the parchment paper out of the pan and cut the granola into bars. Let them cool completely before serving or storing.

Nutrients (per serving)

Calories: 180 kcal Carbohydrates: 22g Fiber: 3g
Protein: 5g Fat: 8g Sugar: 10g Sodium: 70mg
Calcium: 20mg

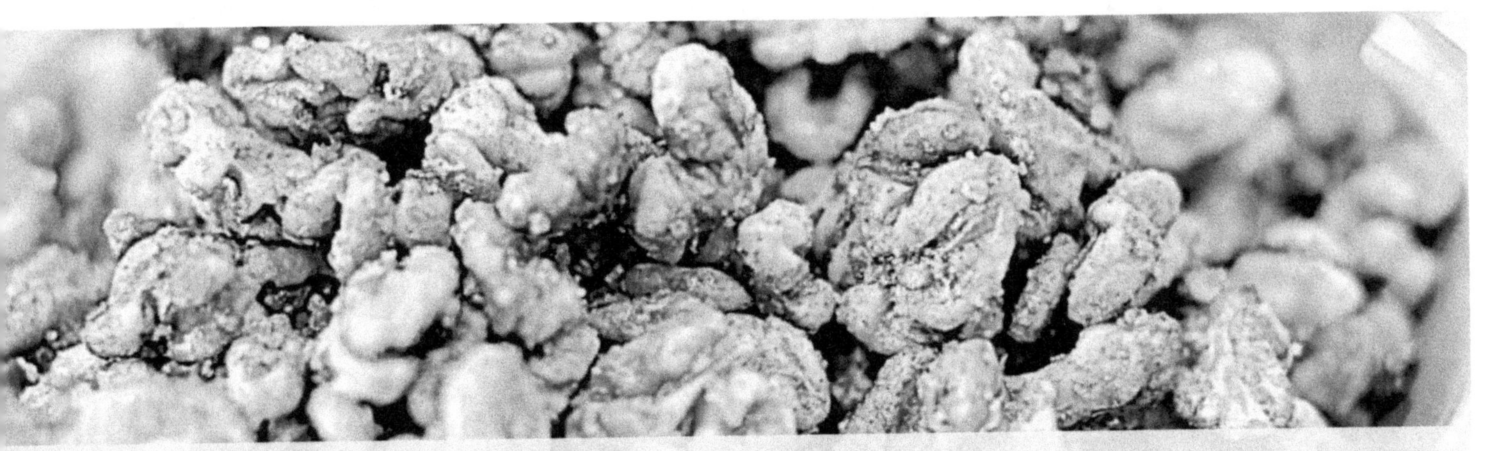

ROASTED WALNUTS WITH SALT

Roasted Walnuts with Salt make for a simple, crunchy, and nutritious snack. They are rich in healthy fats, protein, and antioxidants, providing a perfect energy boost. With just two ingredients, this quick and easy recipe is perfect for healthy snacking, adding to salads, or topping oatmeal.

Serves		Preparation Time		Cooking Time	
4		5 minutes		15 minute	

Ingredients:

2 cups raw walnut halves
1/2 teaspoon sea salt (adjust to taste)

Instructions:

1. **Preheat the Oven:** Preheat your oven to 350°F (175°C).
2. **Prepare the Walnuts:** Spread the walnut halves in a single layer on a baking sheet.
3. **Roast the Walnuts:** Roast the walnuts in the preheated oven for 10-12 minutes, stirring halfway through to ensure even roasting. Keep an eye on them, as they can burn quickly.
4. **Season with Salt:** Remove the walnuts from the oven and immediately sprinkle them with sea salt while they're still hot. Toss the walnuts gently to distribute the salt evenly.
5. **Cool and Serve:** Allow the walnuts to cool completely on the baking sheet. Once cooled, transfer them to an airtight container for storage.

Nutrients (per serving)

Calories: 200 kcal Carbohydrates: 4g Fiber: 2g

Protein: 5g Fat: 20g Sugar: 1g Sodium: 150mg

Calcium: 30mg

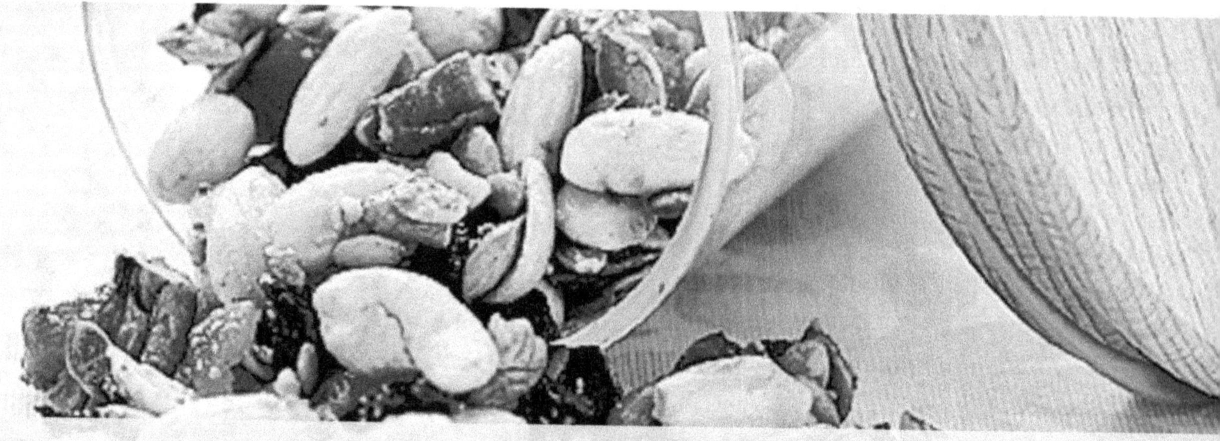

DRIED FRUIT AND NUT MIX

This Dried Fruit and Nut Mix is a perfect on-the-go snack that combines the natural sweetness of dried fruits with the crunchy texture of nuts. Packed with healthy fats, fiber, and essential nutrients, it's a balanced and energizing option for a quick snack, hiking trip, or even as a topping for yogurt or salads.

Serves	 Preparation Time	 Cooking Time	
4	5 minutes	0 minute	

Ingredients:

1/2 cup almonds
1/2 cup walnuts
1/2 cup cashews
1/4 cup dried cranberries
1/4 cup dried apricots, chopped
1/4 cup raisins
1/4 cup dried blueberries

Instructions:

1. **Combine the Ingredients:** In a large bowl, combine the almonds, walnuts, cashews, dried cranberries, dried apricots, raisins, and dried blueberries.
2. **Mix Well:** Gently stir the mixture to ensure all the dried fruits and nuts are evenly distributed.
3. **Store:** Store the mix in an airtight container at room temperature. It will stay fresh for up to two weeks.
4. **Serve:** Enjoy the mix as a snack on its own, or sprinkle it over yogurt, oatmeal, or salads for extra flavor and texture.

Nutrients (per serving)

Calories: 250 kcal Carbohydrates: 22g Fiber: 4g

Protein: 6g Fat: 16g Sugar: 16g Sodium: 10mg

Calcium: 40mg

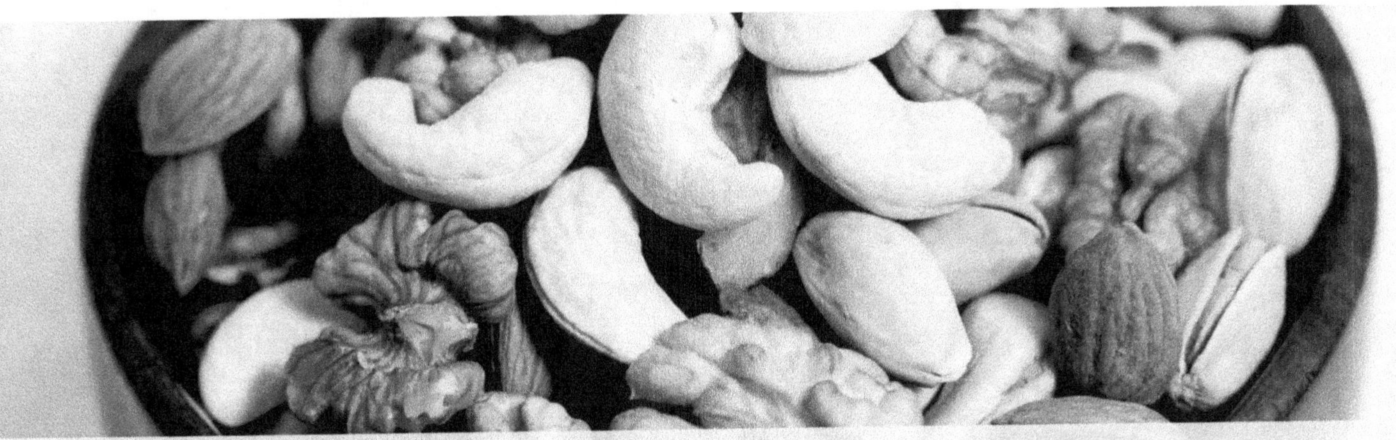

ALMONDS AND PISTACHIOS SNACK

This Almonds and Pistachios Snack is a simple, yet highly nutritious and flavorful option for anyone seeking a quick bite. Combining the nutty richness of almonds and the slightly sweet, buttery flavor of pistachios, this snack is packed with healthy fats, protein, and fiber, making it an excellent choice for curbing hunger between meals.

Serves	 Preparation Time	 Cooking Time 
4	5 minutes	0 minute

Ingredients:

1/2 cup raw almonds
1/2 cup shelled pistachios
1/4 teaspoon sea salt (optional)
1/4 teaspoon ground cinnamon (optional, for a sweet twist)

Instructions:

1. **Combine Nuts:** In a large mixing bowl, combine the raw almonds and shelled pistachios.
2. **Season (Optional):** For added flavor, sprinkle with sea salt and ground cinnamon, then mix well to ensure the seasoning evenly coats the nuts.
3. **Store:** Store the mixture in an airtight container. It can stay fresh for up to two weeks at room temperature or longer if refrigerated.
4. **Serve:** Enjoy as a standalone snack or as part of a trail mix.

Nutrients (per serving)

Calories: 190 kcal Carbohydrates: 8g Fiber: 4g

Protein: 6g Fat: 16g Sugar: 2g Sodium: 50mg

Calcium: 40mg

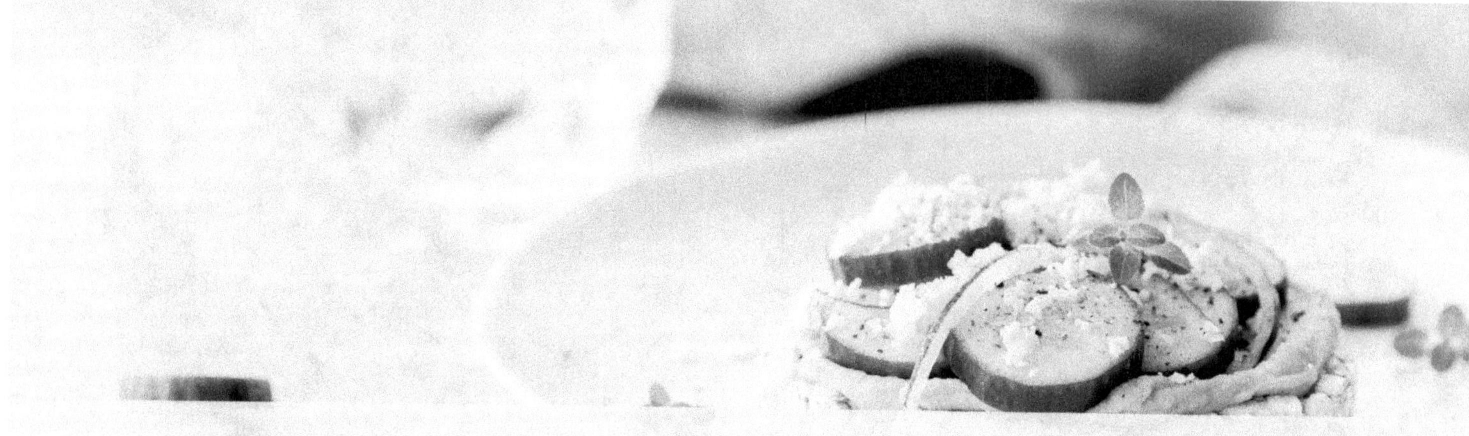

BROWN RICE CRACKERS WITH HUMMUS

Brown Rice Crackers with Hummus is a light yet fulfilling snack, perfect for those looking to combine a crunchy, whole-grain base with the creamy richness of hummus. Packed with fiber and protein, this snack is both nutritious and delicious, ideal for mid-day munching or as an appetizer.

Serves		**Preparation Time**		**Cooking Time**	
4		10 minutes		0 minute	

Ingredients:

16 brown rice crackers (about 4 per person)
1 cup hummus (store-bought or homemade)
1 tablespoon olive oil (optional, for drizzling)
1 teaspoon paprika or cumin (optional, for garnish)
Fresh parsley (optional, for garnish)

Instructions:

1. **Arrange Crackers:** Place 4 brown rice crackers on each plate, evenly spaced.
2. **Prepare Hummus:** If using store-bought hummus, stir it to ensure a smooth texture. For added flavor, drizzle with olive oil and sprinkle paprika or cumin on top.
3. **Serve with Garnish:** Optionally, garnish the hummus with fresh parsley for an extra touch of color and flavor.
4. **Dip and Enjoy:** Serve the hummus alongside the brown rice crackers. Each person can dip or spread the hummus onto the crackers.

Nutrients (per serving)

Calories: 200 kcal Carbohydrates: 24g Fiber: 4g
Protein: 6g Fat: 8g Sugar: 1g Sodium: 150mg
Calcium: 40mg

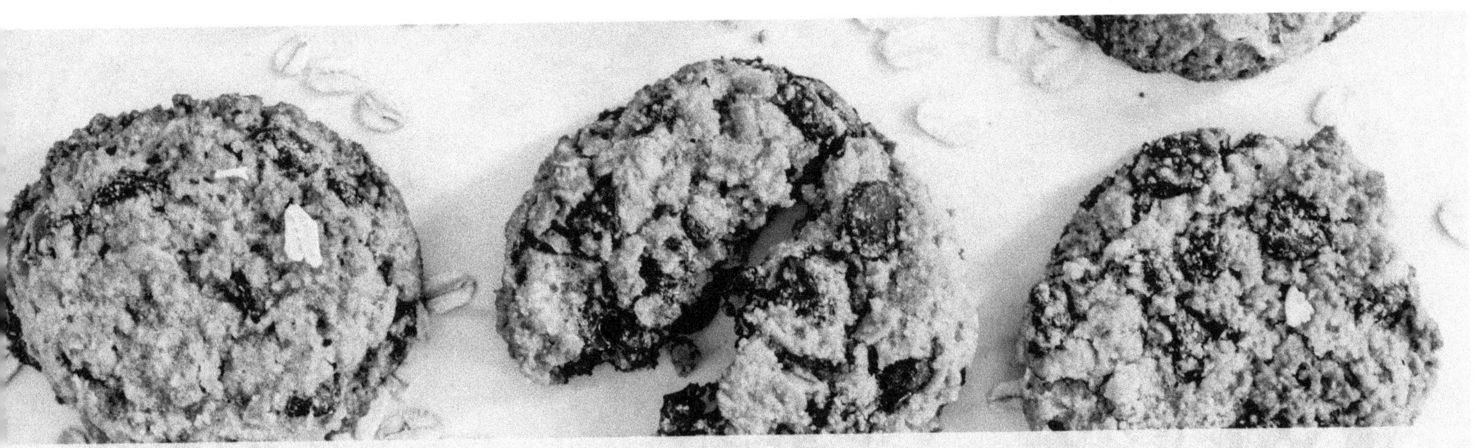

SUGAR-FREE OATMEAL COOKIES

These Sugar-Free Oatmeal Cookies are the perfect healthy treat for anyone looking to enjoy a sweet snack without the added sugar. Made with sucralose and wholesome ingredients like oats and raisins, these cookies are both chewy and satisfying. Great for breakfast, dessert, or an on-the-go snack, they're a guilt-free indulgence.

Serves		**Preparation Time**		**Cooking Time**	
12		10 minutes	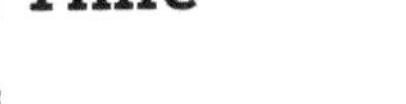	15 minute	

Ingredients:

- 1 1/2 cups rolled oats
- 1/2 cup whole wheat flour
- 1/2 teaspoon baking soda
- 1/2 teaspoon cinnamon
- 1/4 teaspoon salt
- 1/4 cup unsweetened applesauce
- 1/4 cup melted coconut oil
- 1/4 cup sucralose (granular form)
- 1 egg
- 1 teaspoon vanilla extract
- 1/4 cup raisins (optional)

Instructions:

1. **Preheat the Oven:** Preheat your oven to 350°F (175°C) and line a baking sheet with parchment paper.
2. **Mix Dry Ingredients:** In a large bowl, combine rolled oats, whole wheat flour, baking soda, cinnamon, and salt. Mix well.
3. **Prepare Wet Ingredients:** In another bowl, whisk together applesauce, melted coconut oil, sucralose, egg, and vanilla extract until smooth and well-blended.
4. **Combine:** Gradually add the wet ingredients into the dry ingredients. Stir until well combined. If using raisins, fold them into the batter.
5. **Shape the Cookies:** Scoop out about 2 tablespoons of dough per cookie and place them onto the lined baking sheet. Flatten the cookies slightly with a spoon or your fingers.
6. **Bake:** Bake for 12–15 minutes, or until the cookies are golden brown on the edges. Let them co

Nutrients (per serving)

Calories: 90 kcal Carbohydrates: 12g Fiber: 2g

Protein: 2g Fat: 4g Sugar: 0g (with sucralose)

Sodium: 50mg Calcium: 15mg

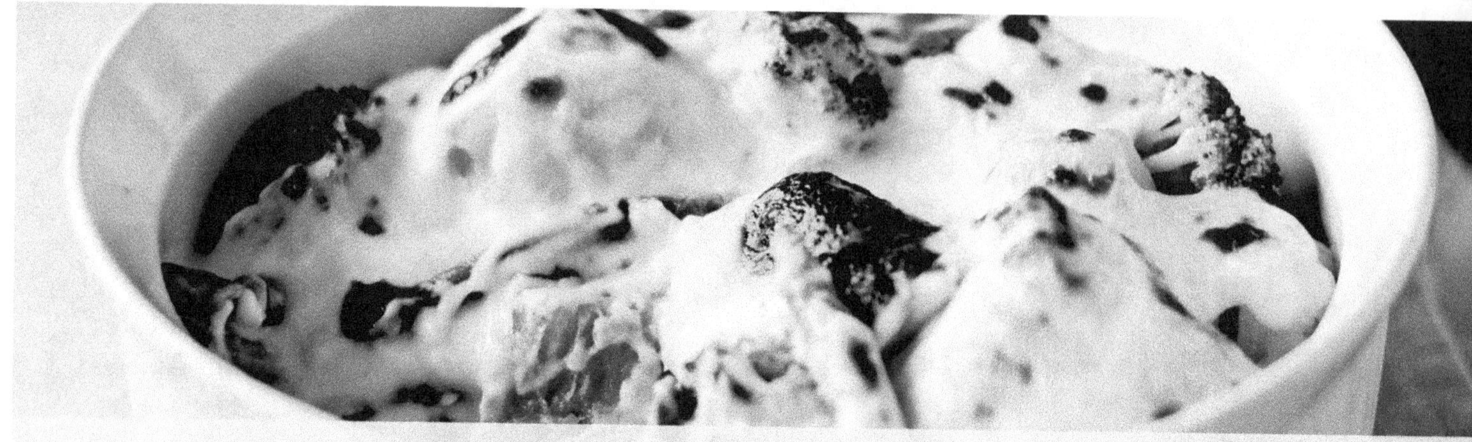

ROASTED VEGETABLES WITH CHEESE DIP

Roasted Vegetables with Cheese Dip is a simple yet flavorful dish, perfect for a healthy snack or side dish. The roasted vegetables, seasoned and caramelized to perfection, are paired with a creamy cheese dip, offering a delightful contrast in texture and flavor. This recipe uses sucralose to add a hint of sweetness to the dip without added sugar, making it a nutritious, low-carb option.

Serves	**Preparation Time**	**Cooking Time**
4	10 minutes	25 minute

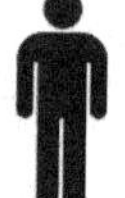

Ingredients:

For Roasted Vegetables:

1 large zucchini, sliced

1 red bell pepper, cut into strips

1 yellow bell pepper, cut into strips

1 red onion, cut into wedges

2 tablespoons olive oil

1/2 teaspoon garlic powder

Salt and pepper to taste

For Cheese Dip:

1/2 cup cream cheese, softened

1/4 cup Greek yogurt

1/4 cup shredded cheddar cheese

1 tablespoon sucralose (granular form)

1/2 teaspoon garlic powder

Salt and pepper to taste

Instructions:

1. **Preheat the Oven:** Preheat your oven to 400°F (200°C) and line a baking sheet with parchment paper.
2. **Prepare Vegetables:** Place the zucchini, bell peppers, and onion on the baking sheet. Drizzle with olive oil, sprinkle with garlic powder, salt, and pepper. Toss to coat evenly.
3. **Roast Vegetables:** Spread the vegetables in a single layer on the baking sheet. Roast for 20-25 minutes, stirring halfway through, until they are tender and lightly browned.
4. **Make the Cheese Dip:** While the vegetables are roasting, prepare the cheese dip. In a bowl, combine cream cheese, Greek yogurt, shredded cheddar, sucralose, garlic powder, salt, and pepper. Stir until smooth and well-mixed.
5. **Serve:** Once the vegetables are roasted, transfer them to a serving platter. Serve with the cheese dip on the side.

Nutrients (per serving)

Calories: 170 kcal Carbohydrates: 7g Fiber: 2g

Protein: 5g Fat: 12g Sugar: 1g Sodium: 250mg

Calcium: 80mg

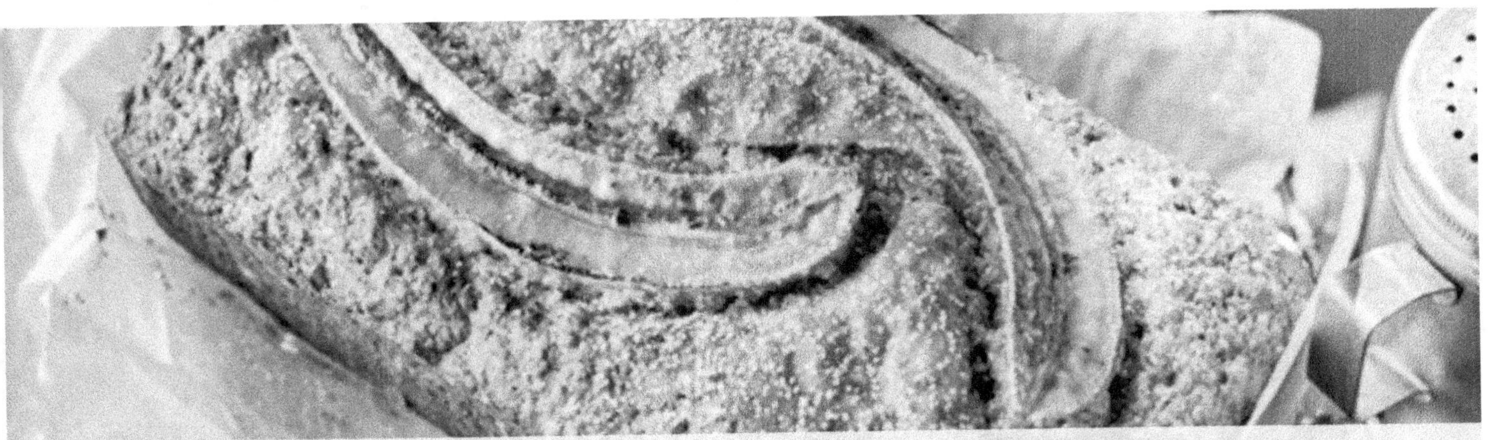

SUGAR-FREE BANANA BREAD

This Sugar-Free Banana Bread is a healthier twist on the classic comfort food, using sucralose as a sugar alternative. It's moist, flavorful, and packed with the natural sweetness of ripe bananas. Perfect for breakfast or as a snack, this banana bread is not only delicious but also suitable for those looking to reduce their sugar intake.

Serves		**Preparation Time**		**Cooking Time**	
8		15 minutes		60 minute	

Ingredients:

3 ripe bananas, mashed

1/3 cup melted coconut oil

1/4 cup sucralose (granular form)

1 teaspoon vanilla extract

2 large eggs

1 1/2 cups whole wheat flour

1 teaspoon baking soda

1/2 teaspoon salt

1/2 teaspoon cinnamon (optional)

1/2 cup chopped walnuts (optional)

Instructions:

1. **Preheat the Oven:** Preheat your oven to 350°F (175°C). Grease a loaf pan or line it with parchment paper.
2. **Prepare the Batter:** In a large bowl, mash the bananas until smooth. Stir in melted coconut oil, sucralose, vanilla extract, and eggs until well combined.
3. **Mix the Dry Ingredients:** In a separate bowl, whisk together the whole wheat flour, baking soda, salt, and cinnamon (if using). Gradually add the dry ingredients into the wet banana mixture, stirring until just combined. Do not overmix.
4. **Fold in Add-Ins (Optional):** Gently fold in chopped walnuts if using.
5. **Bake:** Pour the batter into the prepared loaf pan and smooth the top. Bake for 50-60 minutes, or until a toothpick inserted into the center comes out clean.
6. **Cool and Serve:** Allow the banana bread to cool in the pan for about 10 minutes, then transfer to a wire rack to cool completely before slicing.

Nutrients (per serving)

Calories: 180 kcal Carbohydrates: 23g Fiber: 3g

Protein: 4g Fat: 8g Sugar: 5g (from bananas)

Sodium: 220mg Calcium: 25mg

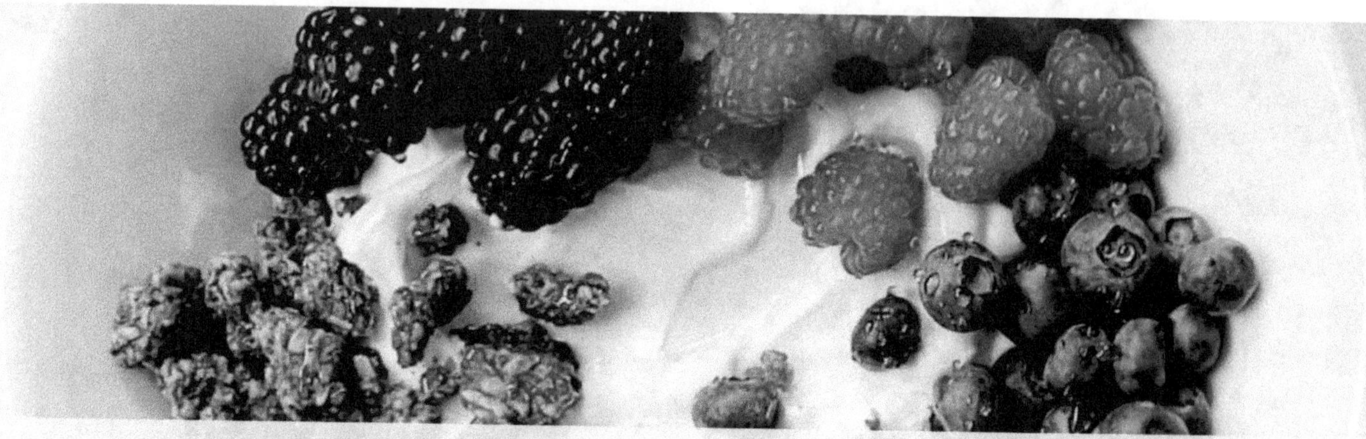

FRESH FRUIT WITH GREEK YOGURT

This Fresh Fruit with Greek Yogurt dish is a light, refreshing, and nutrient-packed snack or breakfast option. The combination of creamy Greek yogurt and naturally sweet, fresh fruits makes it a healthy, protein-rich dish that satisfies hunger and supports balanced nutrition.

Serves		Preparation Time		Cooking Time	
4		10 minutes		0 minute	

Ingredients:

2 cups plain Greek yogurt (unsweetened, low-fat)
1/4 cup sucralose (granular form)
1/2 teaspoon vanilla extract
1 cup strawberries, sliced
1 cup blueberries
1 cup diced kiwi
1/4 cup almonds, chopped (optional)
1 tablespoon chia seeds (optional)

Instructions:

1. **Prepare the Yogurt Base:** In a mixing bowl, combine Greek yogurt, sucralose, and vanilla extract. Stir until well mixed and smooth.
2. **Assemble the Fruit and Yogurt:** Divide the yogurt mixture into four serving bowls.
3. **Add the Fresh Fruit:** Top each bowl with equal portions of sliced strawberries, blueberries, and diced kiwi.
4. **Optional Toppings:** Sprinkle each bowl with chopped almonds and chia seeds for added crunch and nutrition.
5. **Serve:** Serve immediately and enjoy the freshness of the fruit combined with the creamy yogurt.

Nutrients (per serving)

Calories: 140 kcal Carbohydrates: 15g Fiber: 4g
Protein: 10g Fat: 4g Sugar: 7g (from fruit)
Sodium: 60mg Calcium: 120mg

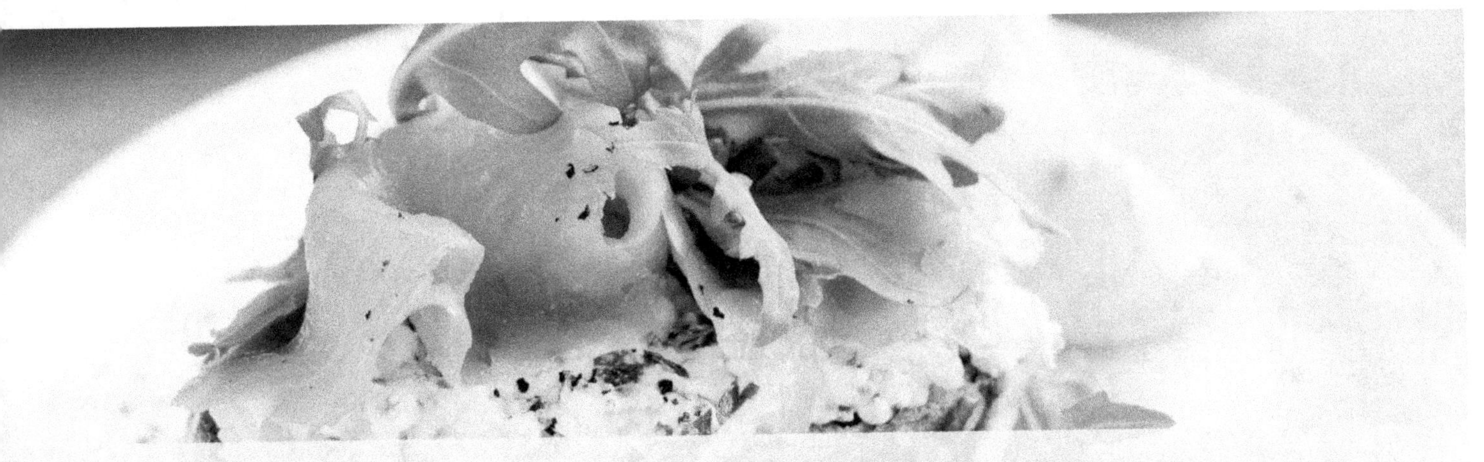

WHOLE WHEAT BREAD WITH COTTAGE CHEESE

Whole Wheat Bread with Cottage Cheese is a simple, nutritious, and satisfying snack or light breakfast. This dish combines the wholesome goodness of whole wheat bread with the creamy texture of cottage cheese, offering a balanced mix of protein, fiber, and healthy carbohydrates.

Serves		Preparation Time		Cooking Time	
4	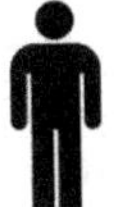	5 minutes		0 minute	

Ingredients:

- 4 slices of whole wheat bread (toasted)
- 1 cup low-fat cottage cheese
- 2 teaspoons sucralose (granular form)
- 1 tablespoon olive oil
- 1 teaspoon black pepper (optional)
- 1 tablespoon fresh herbs (such as chives or parsley, chopped)
- 1/4 cup cherry tomatoes (optional, for garnish)

Instructions:

1. **Prepare the Cottage Cheese Spread:** In a small bowl, mix cottage cheese with sucralose, olive oil, and black pepper until well combined. Adjust the seasoning according to taste.
2. **Toast the Bread:** Toast the whole wheat bread slices until golden brown.
3. **Assemble the Dish:** Spread an even layer of the cottage cheese mixture on each slice of toasted whole wheat bread.
4. **Optional Garnish:** Garnish with fresh herbs and cherry tomatoes for added flavor and color.
5. **Serve:** Serve immediately and enjoy as a healthy snack or breakfast.

Nutrients (per serving)

Calories: 190 kcal Carbohydrates: 22g Fiber: 4g

Protein: 12g Fat: 6g Sugar: 2g Sodium: 350mg

Calcium: 80mg

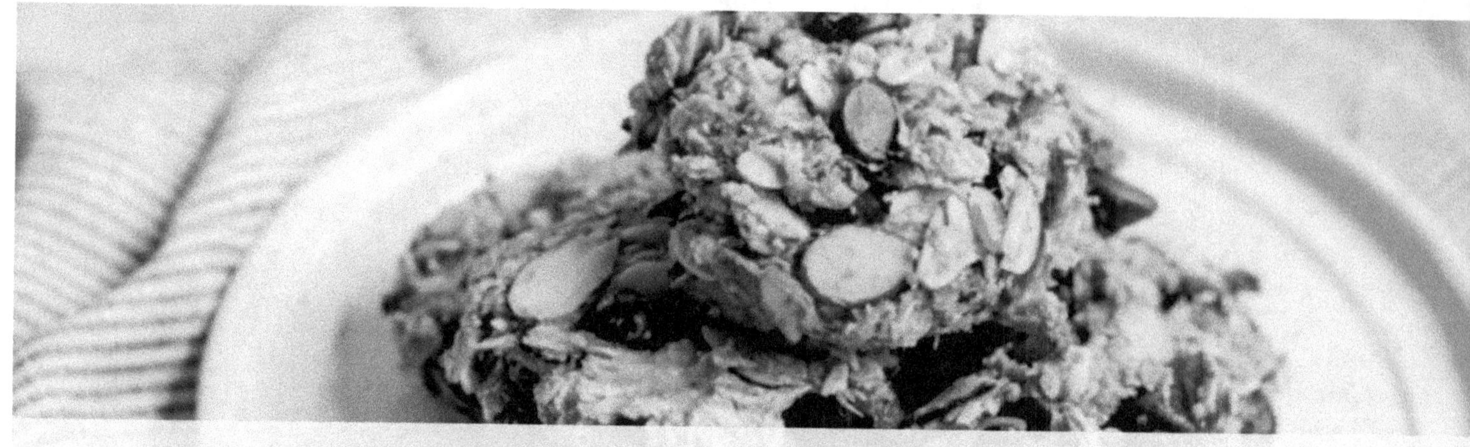

GLUTEN-FREE FLAXSEED COOKIES

Gluten-Free Flaxseed Cookies are a wholesome and delicious treat that caters to those with gluten sensitivities or those simply looking to enjoy a healthy, fiber-rich snack. These cookies are packed with flaxseeds, which provide essential omega-3 fatty acids and fiber, making them a nutritious choice for any time of the day.

Serves 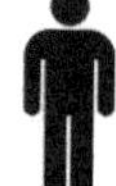	**Preparation Time** 	**Cooking Time** 
12	10 minutes	15 minute

Ingredients:

1 cup almond flour
1/2 cup ground flaxseeds
1/4 cup sucralose (granular form)
1/4 cup coconut oil (melted)
1 large egg
1 teaspoon vanilla extract
1/2 teaspoon baking powder
1/4 teaspoon salt
1/4 cup chopped nuts or dark chocolate chips
(optional)

Instructions:

1. **Preheat Oven:** Preheat your oven to 350°F (175°C) and line a baking sheet with parchment paper.
2. **Mix Dry Ingredients:** In a medium bowl, combine almond flour, ground flaxseeds, sucralose, baking powder, and salt.
3. **Combine Wet Ingredients:** In a separate bowl, whisk together the melted coconut oil, egg, and vanilla extract until well combined.
4. **Form the Dough:** Gradually add the wet ingredients to the dry ingredients, mixing until a dough forms. If using, fold in the chopped nuts or dark chocolate chips.
5. **Shape Cookies:** Scoop tablespoon-sized amounts of dough onto the prepared baking sheet, spacing them about 2 inches apart. Flatten each dough ball slightly with the back of a spoon.
6. **Bake:** Bake in the preheated oven for 12-15 minutes, or until the edges are golden brown.
7. **Cool:** Allow the cookies to cool on the baking sheet for 5 minutes before transferring them to a wire rack to cool completely.

Nutrients (per serving)

Calories: 110 kcal Carbohydrates: 5g Fiber: 3g
Protein: 4g Fat: 9g Sugar: 1g Sodium: 80mg
Calcium: 50mg

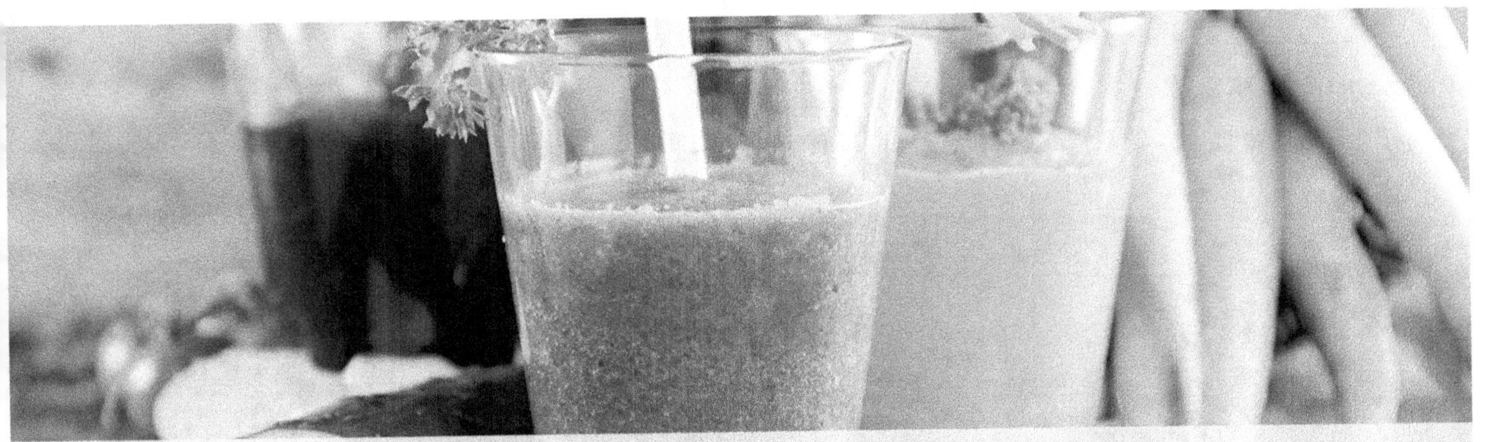

FRUIT AND VEGGIE SMOOTHIE

The Fruit and Veggie Smoothie is a vibrant and nutritious drink that combines the natural sweetness of fruits with the health benefits of vegetables. This smoothie is perfect for a quick breakfast, a post-workout snack, or a refreshing drink throughout the day. It's loaded with vitamins, minerals, and antioxidants to help keep you energized and healthy.

Serves	Preparation Time	Cooking Time
2	10 minutes	0 minute

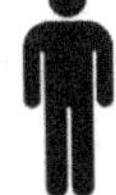  

Ingredients:

1 cup spinach leaves
1/2 cup kale leaves, stems removed
1 medium apple, cored and chopped
1 banana, peeled
1/2 cup frozen berries (such as blueberries, strawberries, or raspberries)
1/2 cup Greek yogurt (plain or vanilla)
1 tablespoon chia seeds
1 tablespoon sucralose (granular form)
1 cup water or unsweetened almond milk
Ice cubes (optional)

Instructions:

1. **Prepare Ingredients:** Wash the spinach and kale thoroughly. Chop the apple into small pieces and peel the banana.
2. **Blend Smoothie:** In a blender, combine the spinach, kale, apple, banana, frozen berries, Greek yogurt, chia seeds, and sucralose.
3. **Add Liquid:** Pour in the water or unsweetened almond milk. If you prefer a colder smoothie, add a few ice cubes.
4. **Blend Until Smooth:** Blend on high speed until all ingredients are well combined and the mixture is smooth. Adjust the consistency by adding more liquid if needed.
5. **Serve:** Pour the smoothie into glasses and serve immediately.

Nutrients (per serving)

Calories: 180 kcal Carbohydrates: 30g Fiber: 6g

Protein: 10g Fat: 2g Sugar: 14g Sodium: 50mg

Calcium: 150mg

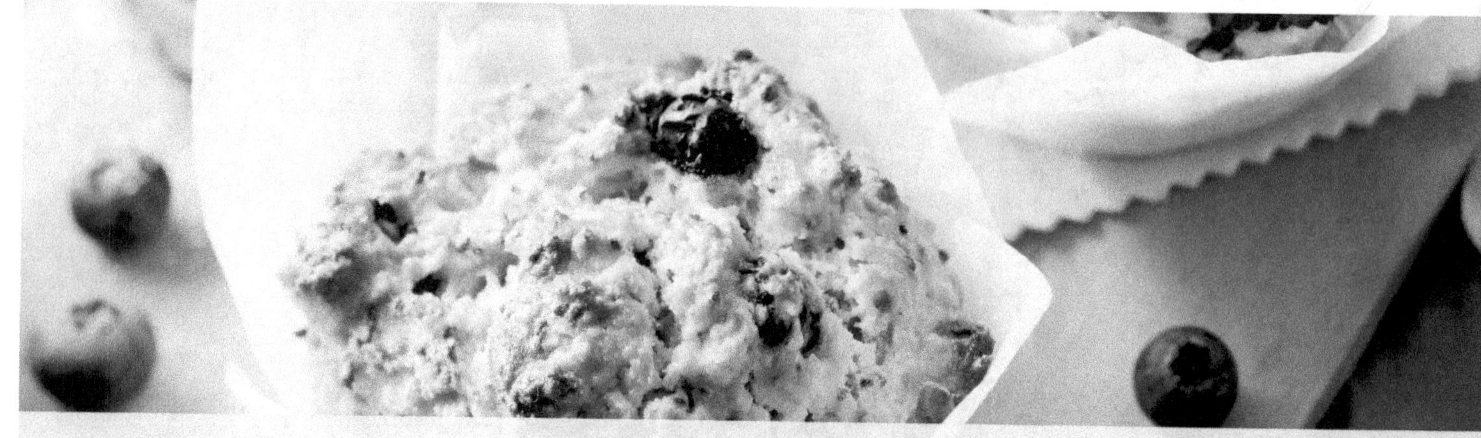

OAT MUFFINS WITH CHIA SEEDS

Oat Muffins with Chia Seeds are a wholesome and nutritious treat perfect for breakfast or a snack. Packed with fiber, protein, and healthy fats, these muffins offer a satisfying and hearty option for those looking to maintain a balanced diet. The combination of oats and chia seeds not only adds a delightful texture but also boosts the nutritional value of these muffins.

Serves		**Preparation Time**		**Cooking Time**	
12		15 minutes		20 minute	

Ingredients:

1 1/2 cups rolled oats

1/2 cup whole wheat flour

1/4 cup chia seeds

1/4 cup sucralose (granular form)

1/2 teaspoon baking powder

1/2 teaspoon baking soda

1/2 teaspoon salt

1/2 teaspoon ground cinnamon

1/2 cup unsweetened applesauce

1/2 cup milk (any kind, including plant-based)

1/4 cup vegetable oil or melted coconut oil

2 large eggs

1 teaspoon vanilla extract

Optional: 1/2 cup blueberries or raisins

Instructions:

1. **Preheat Oven:** Preheat your oven to 350°F (175°C). Line a muffin tin with paper liners or lightly grease it.
2. **Mix Dry Ingredients:** In a large bowl, combine the rolled oats, whole wheat flour, chia seeds, sucralose, baking powder, baking soda, salt, and ground cinnamon. Mix well.
3. **Combine Wet Ingredients:** In another bowl, whisk together the applesauce, milk, oil, eggs, and vanilla extract until well combined.
4. **Combine Wet and Dry Ingredients:** Pour the wet ingredients into the dry ingredients and stir until just combined. If using, fold in the blueberries or raisins.
5. **Fill Muffin Tin:** Divide the batter evenly among the muffin cups, filling each about 3/4 full.
6. **Bake:** Bake in the preheated oven for 18-20 minutes, or until a toothpick inserted into the center of a muffin comes out clean.
7. **Cool and Serve:** Allow the muffins to cool in the tin for 5 minutes before transferring them to a wire rack to cool completely. Serve warm or at room temperature.

Nutrients (per serving)

Calories: 140 kcal Carbohydrates: 17g Fiber: 3g

Protein: 4g Fat: 6g Sugar: 4g Sodium: 150mg

Calcium: 80mg

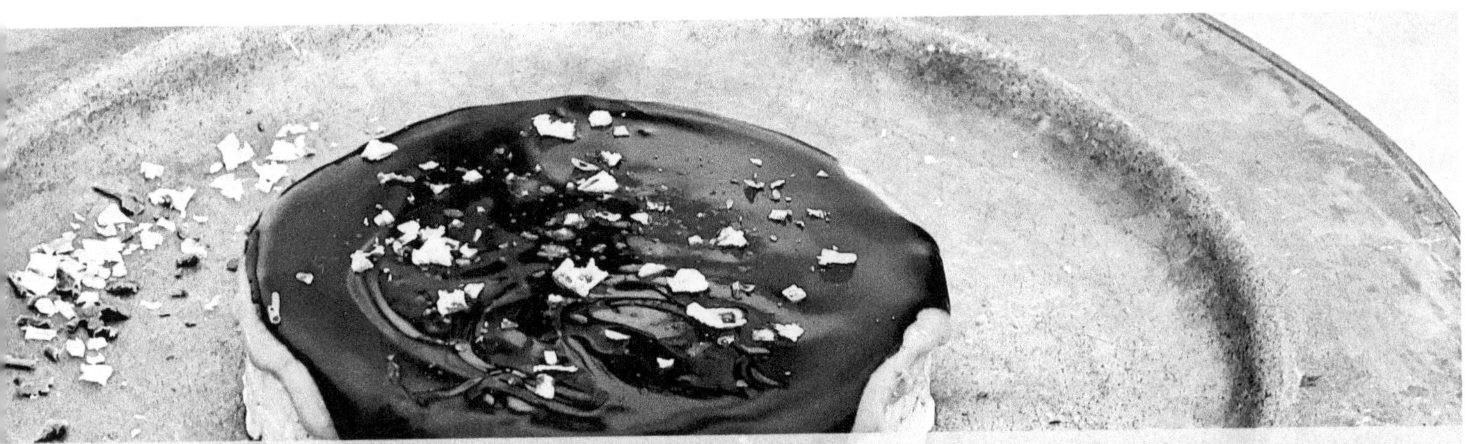

BROWN RICE CAKES WITH PEANUT BUTTER

Brown Rice Cakes with Peanut Butter are a simple yet satisfying snack that combines the crispiness of brown rice cakes with the creamy richness of peanut butter. This snack is not only delicious but also provides a good balance of carbohydrates and protein, making it perfect for a quick energy boost or a light meal. It's an easy-to-make, nutritious option for any time of day.

Serves	Preparation Time	Cooking Time
4	5 minutes	0 minute

Ingredients:

4 brown rice cakes
1/2 cup natural peanut butter
1 tablespoon honey (optional)
1 tablespoon chia seeds (optional)
1/2 banana, sliced (optional)
A sprinkle of cinnamon (optional)

Instructions:

1. **Prepare Peanut Butter:** If desired, mix the natural peanut butter with honey for a touch of sweetness.
2. **Spread Peanut Butter:** Spread an even layer of peanut butter on each brown rice cake.
3. **Add Toppings:** If using, sprinkle chia seeds over the peanut butter. Arrange banana slices on top for added flavor and texture. You can also add a sprinkle of cinnamon if desired.
4. **Serve:** Serve immediately or store in an airtight container for up to 2 days.

Nutrients (per serving)

Calories: 180 kcal Carbohydrates: 17g Fiber: 2g

Protein: 8g Fat: 10g Sugar: 2g Sodium: 150mg

Calcium: 15mg

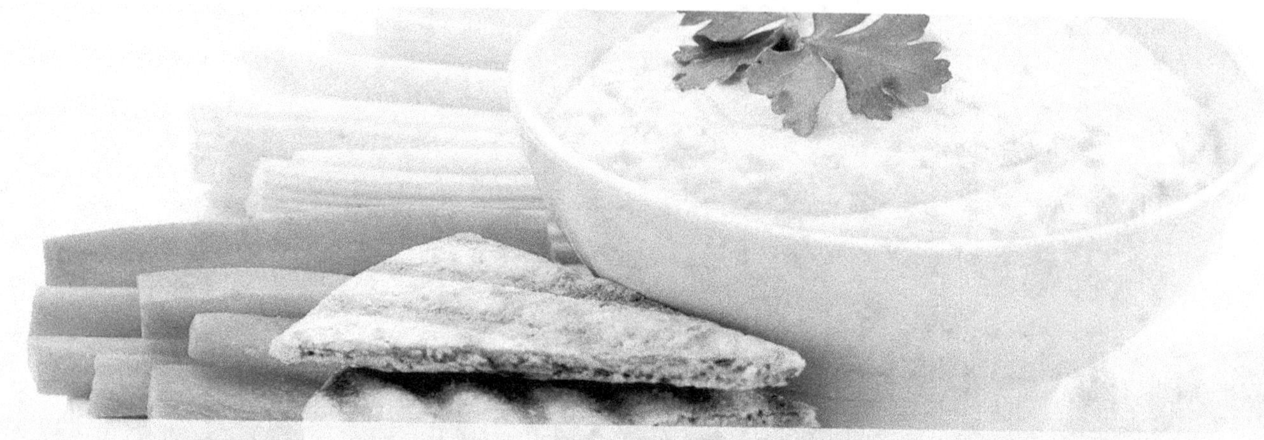

HUMMUS AND CARROT STICKS

Hummus and Carrot Sticks is a classic and nutritious snack that combines the creamy, flavorful goodness of hummus with the crunchy, refreshing bite of fresh carrot sticks. This pairing not only satisfies your taste buds but also provides a healthy dose of fiber, vitamins, and protein. Ideal for a quick snack or a light appetizer, this combo is perfect for anyone looking to enjoy a nutritious, wholesome treat.

Serves 	**Preparation Time**	**Cooking Time** 
4	10 minutes	0 minute

Ingredients:

1 cup hummus (store-bought or homemade)
4 large carrots, peeled and cut into sticks
1 tablespoon olive oil (optional)
1/2 teaspoon paprika (optional)
1/2 teaspoon garlic powder (optional)

Instructions:

1. **Prepare Carrot Sticks:** Peel the carrots and cut them into sticks about 4 inches long and 1/2 inch wide.
2. **Prepare Hummus:** If using store-bought hummus, transfer it to a serving bowl. For homemade hummus, prepare it according to your favorite recipe and place it in a serving bowl.
3. **Season (Optional):** Drizzle olive oil over the hummus, if desired. Sprinkle paprika and garlic powder on top for additional flavor.
4. **Serve:** Arrange the carrot sticks around the bowl of hummus and serve immediately.

Nutrients (per serving)

Calories: 140 kcal Carbohydrates: 14g Fiber: 4g
Protein: 4g Fat: 8g Sugar: 5g Sodium: 200mg
Calcium: 50mg

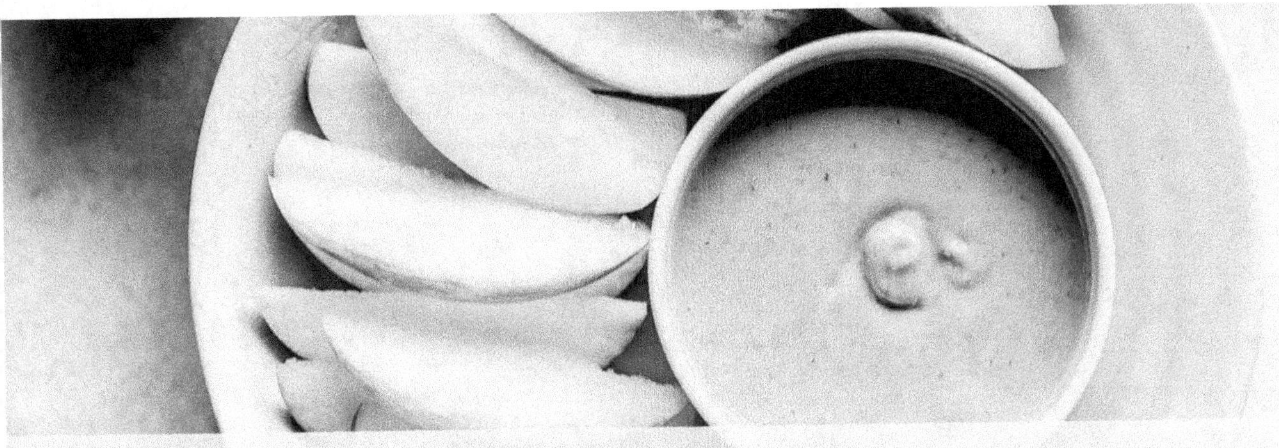

APPLE AND PEANUT BUTTER

Apple and Peanut Butter is a delightful and nutritious snack that combines the crisp, juicy sweetness of apples with the creamy, rich flavor of peanut butter. This pairing offers a satisfying blend of textures and tastes while providing a balanced mix of healthy fats, protein, and fiber. It's perfect for a quick, energizing snack or a light, satisfying treat any time of the day.

Serves		Preparation Time		Cooking Time	
4		5 minutes		0 minute	

Ingredients:

4 medium apples (such as Fuji, Gala, or Honeycrisp)
1/2 cup natural peanut butter (smooth or crunchy)
1 tablespoon honey (optional, for added sweetness)
A pinch of cinnamon (optional, for extra flavor)

Instructions:

1. **Prepare Apples:** Wash and core the apples. Slice them into thin wedges or rounds.
2. **Prepare Peanut Butter:** If desired, stir honey into the peanut butter for added sweetness. You can also sprinkle cinnamon on top of the peanut butter for extra flavor.
3. **Serve:** Arrange apple slices on a plate and serve with a bowl of peanut butter for dipping.

Nutrients (per serving)

Calories: 210 kcal Carbohydrates: 25g Fiber: 5g

Protein: 6g Fat: 11g Sugar: 15g Sodium: 150mg

Calcium: 30mg.

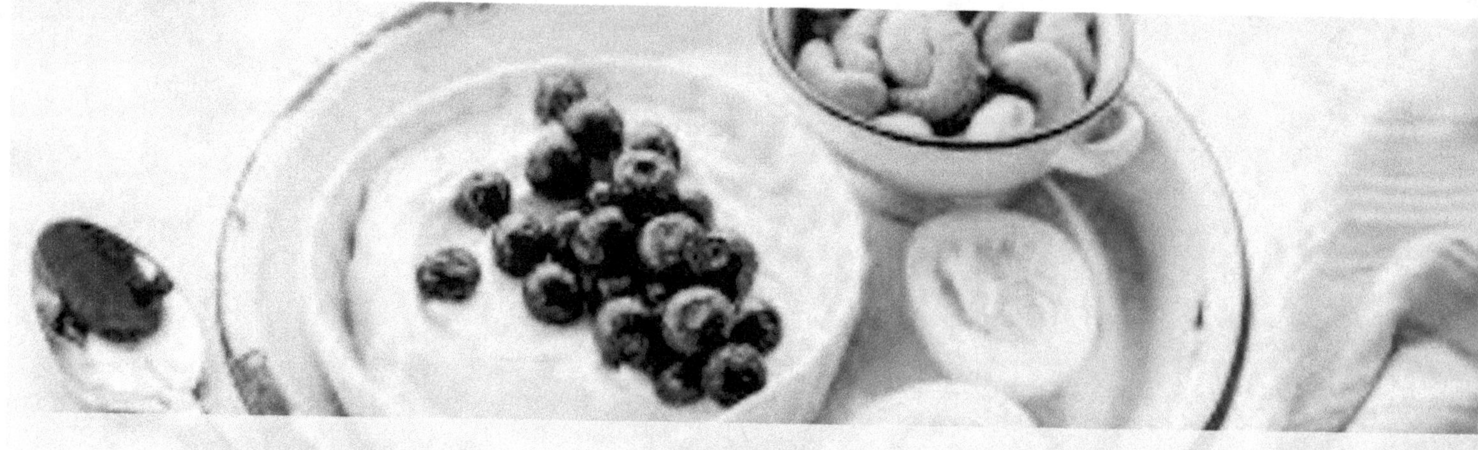

HARD-BOILED EGGS AND CASHEWS

Hard-Boiled Eggs and Cashews is a nutritious and convenient snack pairing that combines the protein-packed goodness of hard-boiled eggs with the crunchy, rich flavor of cashews. This combination offers a satisfying mix of textures and a balance of essential nutrients, making it an ideal choice for a quick snack or a light meal.

Serves	 **Preparation Time**		**Cooking Time**	
4	5 minutes		10 minute	

Ingredients:

1 package (about 2 oz) of dried seaweed sheets (nori)

1 tablespoon olive oil

1/2 teaspoon sea salt

1/2 teaspoon sesame seeds (optional, for garnish)

1/4 teaspoon garlic powder (optional, for added flavor)

Instructions:

1. **Preheat Oven:** Preheat your oven to 300°F (150°C).
2. **Prepare Seaweed:** Place the dried seaweed sheets on a baking sheet lined with parchment paper.Brush each sheet lightly with olive oil.
3. **Season:** Sprinkle sea salt evenly over the seaweed sheets.If using, sprinkle sesame seeds and garlic powder for extra flavor.
4. **Bake:** Bake in the preheated oven for about 8-10 minutes, or until the seaweed sheets are crispy and slightly browned. Keep an eye on them to prevent burning.
5. **Cool:** Remove from the oven and let cool. The seaweed will become crispier as it cools.
6. **Serve:** Break the seaweed sheets into bite-sized pieces and serve as a snack.

Nutrients (per serving)

Calories: 30 kcal Carbohydrates: 1g Fiber: 1g

Protein: 1g Fat: 2g Sugar: 0g Sodium: 150mg

Calcium: 30mg

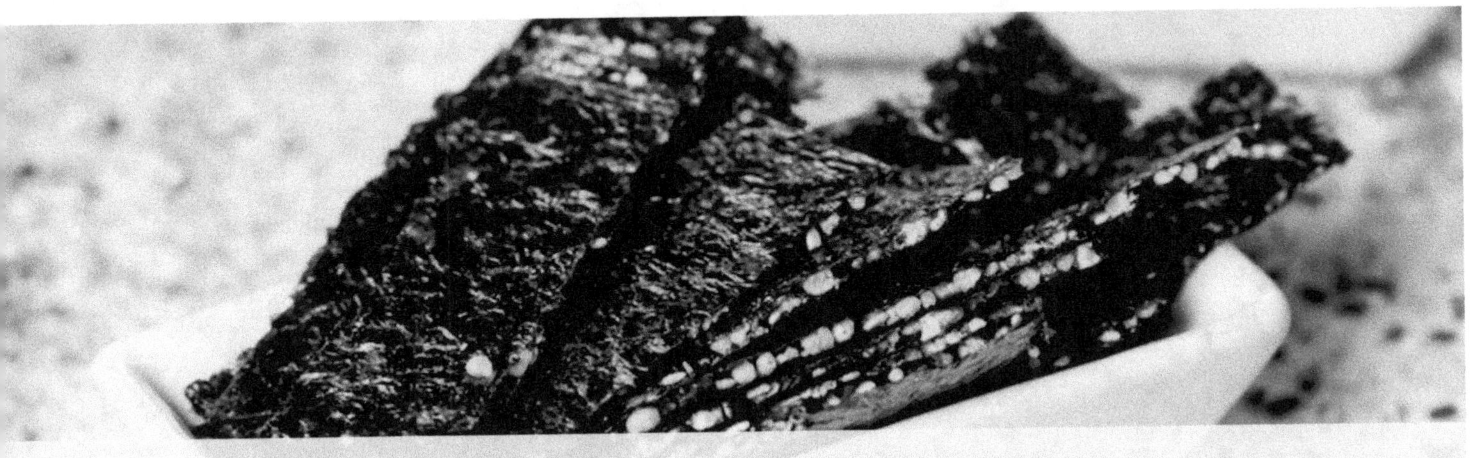

DRIED SEAWEED SNACKS

Dried Seaweed Snacks offer a crispy, savory treat that's both nutritious and satisfying. Rich in essential vitamins and minerals, including iodine and vitamin K, these snacks are a perfect low-calorie option for those looking to add more greens to their diet. Easy to prepare and enjoy, dried seaweed snacks are ideal for on-the-go snacking or as a light, flavorful addition to meals.

Serves		Preparation Time		Cooking Time	
4		10 minutes		10 minute	

Ingredients:

8 large eggs
1/2 cup cashews (unsalted)
A pinch of salt (optional, for seasoning)
A pinch of black pepper (optional, for seasoning)

Instructions:

1. **Boil the Eggs:** Place the eggs in a saucepan and cover them with water. Bring the water to a boil over medium-high heat. Once boiling, reduce the heat to low and let the eggs simmer for 9-10 minutes. Remove the eggs from the hot water and place them in an ice bath to cool.
2. **Prepare the Cashews:** If using raw cashews, toast them lightly in a dry skillet over medium heat for 3-4 minutes, stirring frequently until golden brown. Let them cool.
3. **Serve:** Peel the cooled hard-boiled eggs and cut them in halves or quarters. Arrange the eggs and cashews on a plate. Season the eggs with a pinch of salt and black pepper if desired.

Nutrients (per serving)

Calories: 240 kcal Carbohydrates: 8g Fiber: 1g

Protein: 14g Fat: 18g Sugar: 1g Sodium: 150mg

Calcium: 40mg

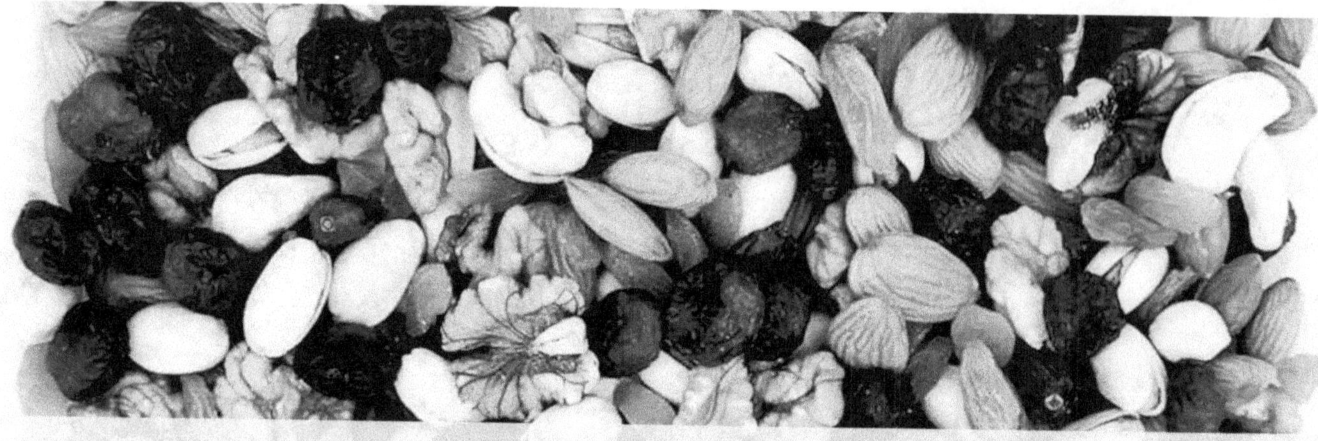

PISTACHIOS AND DRIED FRUIT MIX

Pistachios and Dried Fruit Mix is a delightful combination of crunchy pistachios and naturally sweet dried fruits. This snack blend provides a perfect balance of texture and taste while delivering essential nutrients, including healthy fats, fiber, and vitamins. It's a convenient, portable option for a quick energy boost and a wholesome snack.

Serves 	**Preparation Time**	**Cooking Time** 
4	5 minutes	0 minute

Ingredients:

1 cup raw pistachios (shelled)
1 cup mixed dried fruits (e.g., apricots, raisins, cranberries, or dates)
1/4 cup unsweetened coconut flakes (optional)
1 tablespoon honey or maple syrup (optional, for added sweetness)

Instructions:

1. **Prepare Ingredients:** If the pistachios are not shelled, shell them and set aside.Chop larger dried fruits (such as apricots or dates) into bite-sized pieces if needed.
2. **Mix:** In a large bowl, combine the pistachios and mixed dried fruits.If using, add unsweetened coconut flakes for extra texture and flavor.
3. **Sweeten (Optional):** If you prefer a sweeter mix, drizzle with honey or maple syrup and toss to coat evenly.
4. **Serve:** Divide the mixture into snack-sized portions and serve.

Nutrients (per serving)

Calories: 150 kcal Carbohydrates: 15g Fiber: 3g
Protein: 5g Fat: 8g Sugar: 9g Sodium: 0mg
Calcium: 20mg

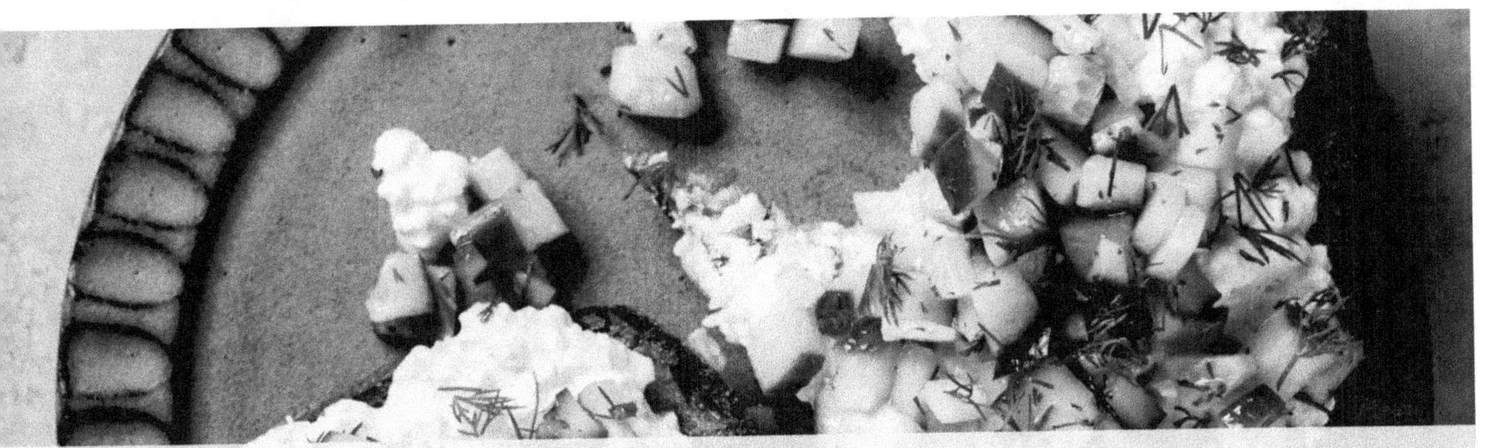

COTTAGE CHEESE AND CUCUMBER

Cottage Cheese and Cucumber is a refreshing and nutritious snack that combines creamy cottage cheese with the crispness of cucumber. This simple yet satisfying dish offers a boost of protein and hydration, making it a perfect light snack or addition to any meal. It's low in calories and packed with essential nutrients, ideal for those seeking a healthy option.

Serves		Preparation Time		Cooking Time	
4		10 minutes		0 minute	

Ingredients:

2 cups cottage cheese (low-fat or full-fat, as desired)
1 large cucumber
1 tablespoon fresh dill (optional, for garnish)
Salt and pepper to taste
1 tablespoon lemon juice (optional)

Instructions:

1. **Prepare the Cucumber:** Wash the cucumber thoroughly. Slice the cucumber into thin rounds or half-moons, depending on preference.
2. **Mix:** In a large bowl, combine the cottage cheese with the sliced cucumber.
3. **Season:** Add salt and pepper to taste. If desired, drizzle with lemon juice for a tangy flavor.
4. **Garnish (Optional):** Sprinkle fresh dill over the top for added freshness and flavor.
5. **Serve:** Divide the mixture into serving bowls and enjoy.

Nutrients (per serving)

Calories: 110 kcal Carbohydrates: 7g Fiber: 1g

Protein: 12g Fat: 4g Sugar: 4g Sodium: 300mg

Calcium: 150mg

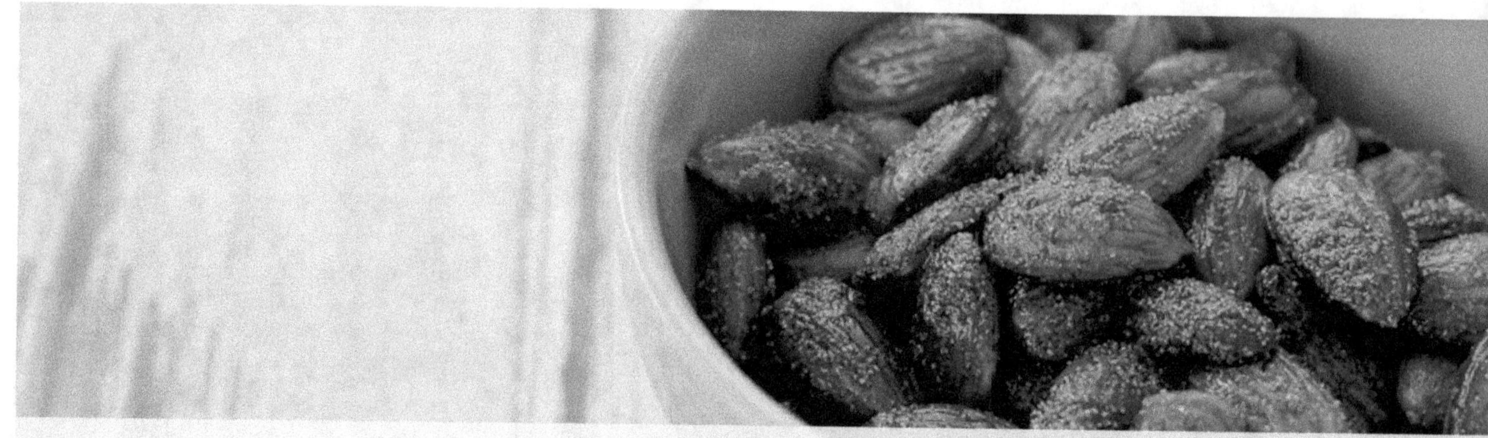

BUTTER ROASTED ALMONDS

Butter Roasted Almonds are a delectable snack that features almonds roasted to perfection with a rich, buttery flavor. This easy-to-make treat is perfect for satisfying cravings, adding a crunchy element to meals, or serving as a flavorful party snack. The combination of roasted almonds and a hint of butter creates a savory snack with a touch of elegance.

Serves		**Preparation Time**		**Cooking Time**	
4		10 minutes		15 minute	

Ingredients:

2 cups raw almonds
2 tablespoons unsalted butter
1/2 teaspoon salt
1/4 teaspoon garlic powder (optional)
1/4 teaspoon paprika (optional)

Instructions:

1. **Preheat Oven:** Preheat your oven to 350°F (175°C).
2. **Prepare Almonds:** Spread the raw almonds evenly on a baking sheet.
3. **Roast Almonds:** Roast the almonds in the preheated oven for 10-12 minutes, or until they are golden and fragrant. Stir once halfway through to ensure even roasting.
4. **Melt Butter:** While the almonds are roasting, melt the unsalted butter in a small saucepan over low heat.
5. **Toss Almonds:** Once the almonds are roasted, remove them from the oven and immediately toss them in the melted butter.
6. **Season:** Sprinkle salt over the almonds. If using, add garlic powder and paprika for extra flavor. Toss to coat evenly.
7. **Cool:** Allow the almonds to cool on the baking sheet for about 5 minutes. They will continue to crisp up as they cool.
8. **Serve:** Transfer the cooled almonds to a serving bowl and enjoy.

Nutrients (per serving)

Calories: 200 kcal Carbohydrates: 7g Fiber: 4g
Protein: 6g Fat: 18g Sugar: 1g Sodium: 150mg
Calcium: 60mg

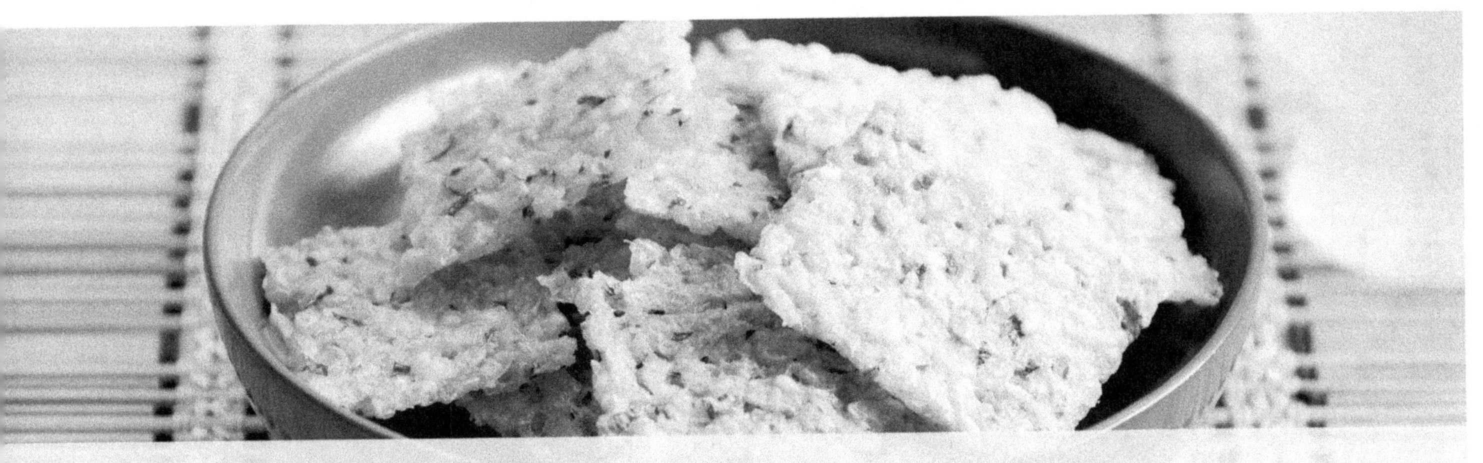

RICE CRACKERS WITH CHEESE

Rice Crackers with Cheese is a simple yet satisfying snack that combines the crispy texture of rice crackers with the creamy richness of cheese. This quick and easy recipe is perfect for a light snack, appetizer, or even a party treat. With minimal preparation and a delightful blend of flavors, this snack is sure to please cheese lovers and those seeking a crunchy, savory treat.

Serves	Preparation Time	Cooking Time
4	5 minutes	5 minute

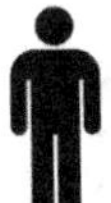  

Ingredients:

1 cup rice crackers
4 ounces cheese (such as cheddar, gouda, or your preferred cheese), sliced or shredded
1 tablespoon fresh herbs (such as chives or parsley), finely chopped (optional)
1/4 teaspoon black pepper (optional)

Instructions:

1. **Prepare Cheese:** Slice or shred the cheese into small pieces that will fit comfortably on the rice crackers.
2. **Arrange Crackers:** Place the rice crackers on a baking sheet or oven-safe plate.
3. **Top with Cheese:** Place a slice or a small amount of shredded cheese on each rice cracker.
4. **Melt Cheese:** Preheat the oven to 350°F (175°C). Bake the crackers with cheese for 3-5 minutes, or until the cheese is melted and bubbly. Keep an eye on them to prevent burning.
5. **Season (Optional):** If desired, sprinkle finely chopped fresh herbs and black pepper on top of the melted cheese.
6. **Cool:** Remove from the oven and let the crackers cool slightly before serving.
7. **Serve:** Arrange the rice crackers with cheese on a serving platter and enjoy.

Nutrients (per serving)

Calories: 150 kcal Carbohydrates: 15g Fiber: 1g
Protein: 6g Fat: 8g Sugar: 1g Sodium: 250mg
Calcium: 150mg

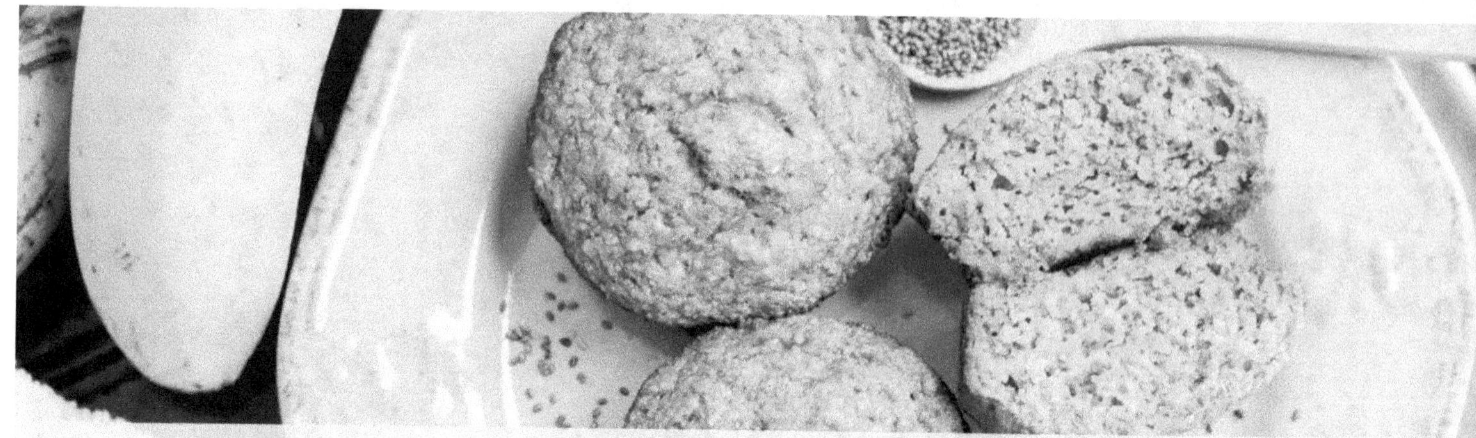

BANANA AND CHIA SEED MUFFINS

Banana and Chia Seed Muffins are a wholesome and delicious treat that combines the natural sweetness of ripe bananas with the nutritional benefits of chia seeds. These muffins are perfect for breakfast or a snack and are packed with fiber, omega-3 fatty acids, and essential nutrients. They are easy to make and provide a satisfying, guilt-free indulgence.

Serves		**Preparation Time**		**Cooking Time**	
12		10 minutes		25 minute	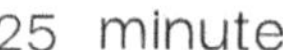

Ingredients:

1 1/2 cups all-purpose flour
1/2 cup chia seeds
1/2 teaspoon baking soda
1/2 teaspoon baking powder
1/4 teaspoon salt
1/2 cup brown sugar
1/4 cup unsweetened applesauce
2 large ripe bananas, mashed
1/4 cup vegetable oil or melted coconut oil
2 large eggs
1 teaspoon vanilla extract
1/2 cup chopped walnuts or pecans (optional)

Instructions:

1. **Preheat Oven:** Preheat your oven to 350°F (175°C). Line a 12-cup muffin tin with paper liners or lightly grease it.
2. **Mix Dry Ingredients:** In a medium bowl, whisk together the flour, chia seeds, baking soda, baking powder, and salt.
3. **Combine Wet Ingredients:** In a large bowl, mix the brown sugar, applesauce, mashed bananas, oil, eggs, and vanilla extract until well combined.
4. **Combine Mixtures:** Gradually add the dry ingredients to the wet ingredients, stirring until just combined. Do not overmix. If using, fold in the chopped walnuts or pecans.
5. **Fill Muffin Tin:** Divide the batter evenly among the 12 muffin cups, filling each about 2/3 full.
6. **Bake:** Bake in the preheated oven for 20-25 minutes, or until a toothpick inserted into the center of a muffin comes out clean.
7. **Cool:** Allow the muffins to cool in the tin for 5 minutes, then transfer them to a wire rack to cool completely.
8. **Serve:** Enjoy the muffins warm or at room temperature.

Nutrients (per serving)

Calories: 150 kcal Carbohydrates: 20g Fiber: 3g
Protein: 4g Fat: 6g Sugar: 9g Sodium: 180mg
Calcium: 50mg

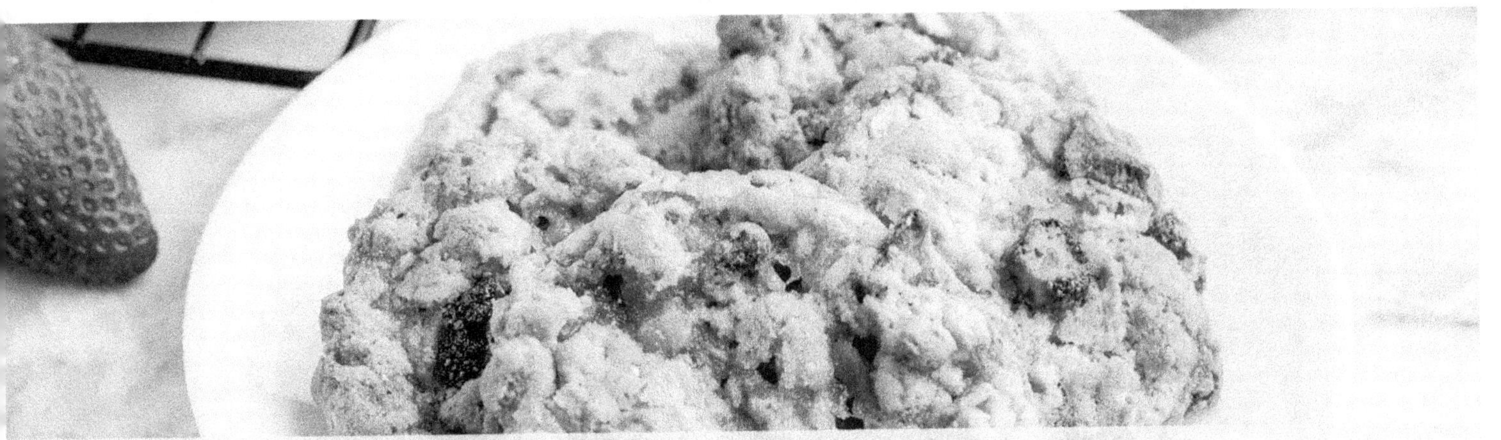

OATMEAL COOKIES WITH STRAWBERRIES

Oatmeal Cookies with Strawberries combine the heartiness of oats with the sweet, juicy flavor of fresh strawberries. These cookies are a delightful treat that balances a satisfying texture with a burst of fruity sweetness. They're perfect for a snack or a light dessert and offer a nutritious twist on traditional cookies.

Serves		**Preparation Time**		**Cooking Time**	
24		15 minutes		15 minute	

Ingredients:

1 cup old-fashioned oats
1/2 cup all-purpose flour
1/2 teaspoon baking powder
1/4 teaspoon baking soda
1/4 teaspoon salt
1/2 cup unsalted butter, softened
1/2 cup brown sugar
1/4 cup granulated sugar
1 large egg
1 teaspoon vanilla extract
1 cup fresh strawberries, chopped
1/4 cup chopped nuts (optional)

Instructions:

1. **Preheat Oven:** Preheat your oven to 350°F (175°C). Line a baking sheet with parchment paper or a silicone baking mat.
2. **Mix Dry Ingredients:** In a medium bowl, combine the oats, flour, baking powder, baking soda, and salt. Stir to mix well.
3. **Cream Butter and Sugars:** In a large bowl, use an electric mixer to beat the softened butter, brown sugar, and granulated sugar until light and fluffy.
4. **Add Wet Ingredients:** Beat in the egg and vanilla extract until well combined.
5. **Combine Mixtures:** Gradually add the dry ingredients to the wet ingredients, mixing just until combined. Gently fold in the chopped strawberries and nuts (if using).
6. **Scoop Dough:** Drop rounded tablespoons of dough onto the prepared baking sheet, spacing them about 2 inches apart.
7. **Bake:** Bake in the preheated oven for 10-12 minutes, or until the edges are golden brown and the centers are set.
8. **Cool:** Allow the cookies to cool on the baking sheet for 5 minutes before transferring them to a wire rack to cool completely.
9. **Serve:** Enjoy the cookies warm or at room temperature.

Nutrients (per serving)

Calories: 110 kcal Carbohydrates: 15g Fiber: 1g

Protein: 2g Fat: 5g Sugar: 8g Sodium: 80mg

Calcium: 20mg